Blood Sı

What You Need T
Optimal Lifestyle Plan For
Preventing Diseases, Diabetes,
Losing Weight & Natural,
Amazing Health

CW00500425

Copyright Notice

Disclaimer

Claim your FREE Audiobook Now

Autoimmune Healing Transform Your Health, Reduce Inflammation, Heal the Immune System and Start Living Healthy
Do you have an overall sense of not feeling your best, but it has been going on so long that it's actually normal to you?
If you answered yes to any of these question, you may have an autoimmune disease.
Autoimmune diseases are one of the ten leading causes of death for women in all age groups and they affect nearly 25 million Americans.
In fact millions of people worldwide suffer from autoimmunity whether they know it or not.

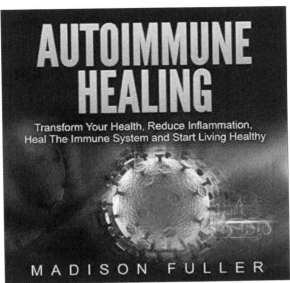

Free Newsletter

Health, longevity and lifestyle tips and advice
Sign up to get the exclusive Madison Fuller e-newsletter, sent out every week

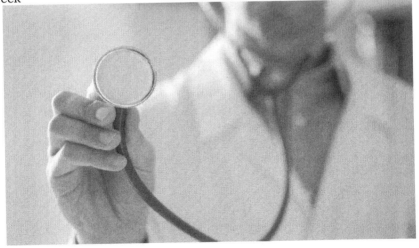

Sign Up

Table of Contents

Introduction

Congratulations on purchasing *Blood Sugar: What You Need To Know, The Optimal Lifestyle Plan For Preventing Diseases, Diabetes, Losing Weight & Natural, Amazing Health,* and thank you for doing so.

Abnormal blood sugars are one of the most serious health problems a person can develop. High blood sugar is closely associated with diabetes, and the damage it can cause throughout the body means that if you have high blood sugar for an extended period of time, you are going to be at risk for developing many health problems. High blood sugar can damage nearly every organ system in the body from the eyes to the heart to the kidneys. Diabetics are at very high risk for developing heart disease, high blood pressure, kidney problems, blindness, and even cancer.

For decades, medical doctors have simply accepted diabetes. The focus has been on managing the disease with pharmaceuticals once people come down with it, rather than on managing it naturally or even preventing it in the first place. This approach has not been all that successful. When attempting to manage the disease with pills and insulin injections, the health of the patient gradually worsens over time. Higher and higher doses of medications become necessary, and eventually, they may not work at all. The patient is then forced to live a life that centers on constant injections of insulin, making day to day existence and never-ending battle. There are always risks of having blood sugar go too high, or having it drop too low by accidentally injecting too much insulin.

Even when the patient is able to manage it properly, the pain and difficulty of having to use insulin injections to lead a seemingly normal life becomes overwhelming. And even then, health will continue to worsen in many patients.

If you want to live a life of having to constantly worry while being completely dependent on drugs and insulin injections and facing worsening health over time, you can follow the conventional approach. But these days, more and more people with blood sugar problems are taking control of their own health. Many of them are even throwing away their medications and using completely natural means of managing and even reversing their diabetes. The good news is that you can do that too, and we will be showing you some of the ways you can do it in this book.

You may be experiencing your own problems with high blood sugar and even diabetes right now. And you may have had friends and relatives who've dealt with these problems. In my own life, I've had many friends that succumbed to the disease. Some friends were not that diligent about keeping up with their medications and insulin injections. As a result, they ended up with major health problems. One man I knew developed several sores on his leg that wouldn't heal, and they ended up having to amputate it. He ended up dying at a young age and spent his last years suffering.

I have a history of diabetes in my own family. My mother was diabetic, and I saw what it did to her. Although she lived a long life, she was dependent on insulin and drugs for several decades. When you're in that situation, you can't just sit down and eat a meal, especially if it's something like a birthday celebration where people might have cake or other sweets like ice cream. She had to constantly stay on top of her insulin injections, taking the daily medications, and doing everything at just the right time, centered around her meals. And despite all that diligence and living an active life with lots of exercise, she developed many of the complications that result from the disease. This included needed a triple bypass in order to reduce the risk of getting a heart attack, and problems with her eyesight that led to partial blindness.

Naturally, given the hereditary tendencies of the disease, I was always worried about it. And over the years, my weight crept up, and so did my blood sugars. Soon, I was solidly in the prediabetic range (I will be telling you what that is in the book). Despite following standard recommendations and doing some exercise, I developed high blood pressure, and my blood sugar readings kept going higher and higher until finally they were in the diabetic range.

At that point, my doctors gave me one last chance. If I didn't succeed, they were going to put me on medications. So I dove into the research and found out the latest discoveries on diet, lifestyle, and exercise that could help reverse diabetes. Within six months, the trends in my blood sugars had begun reversing, and pretty soon they were back to normal levels.

If you are having blood sugar problems, you must act on this immediately. If you don't, your health will continue to worsen, and with every passing day that you have high blood sugar, you are damaging blood vessels throughout the body and the organs you feed. As we will see, high blood sugars can even feed cancer cells, leading to the development of dangerous tumors. But you can avoid all this – by changing your lifestyle now.

I will be sharing some of the secrets I discovered in this book, and I will show you how to apply them in your own life. You can take control of your own health and avoid the medications and insulin injections, along with worsening health that comes with diabetes. It does take some discipline, but I promise that any reader who changes their lifestyle can prevent or even reverse diabetes. In doing so, you will significantly reduce the risk of developing many diseases and conditions.

I urge all readers to at least try taking control of their own health and blood sugar by following the methods laid out in this book. If you are on medication, be sure to inform your doctor of any lifestyle changes, so they can adjust your medication if necessary and keep a close eye on your health.

There are plenty of books on this subject on the market, thanks again for choosing this one! Every effort was made to ensure it is full of as much useful information as possible; please enjoy!

Chapter 1: High Blood Sugar: What It Does to the Body

In this chapter, we are going to get into the details of what blood sugar is and what high blood sugars do to the body. In the modern world, where many infectious diseases and other conditions have been made easily curable, high blood sugar has moved to the forefront of major health problems. This is also a problem that comes about because more people are living longer and dealing with the problems of obesity or being overweight.

In this chapter, we are going to discuss what blood sugar is. In order to understand this, we will need to discuss how your body gets energy, and the different ways that energy is stored in plants and other food items, and the basic way that your body is able to get energy out of the food that we eat.

We will also discuss diabetes and complications of high blood sugar. Then we will look at the role that the food industry, medical establishment, and big pharmaceutical companies are playing in the ongoing epidemic.

What is Blood Sugar?

Blood sugar is simply sugar that is present in your bloodstream. It gets there from the food you eat, specifically from the fruit, vegetables, and breads and pastas that you consume. Even if you didn't consume any of those foods, you would still have blood sugar, because certain cells in your body need sugar in order to survive. The sugar in your blood provides the energy that your body needs to function.

There are two ways that your body can derive energy. You can get energy from fat or from sugar. When you get energy from fat, the fat is broken down into molecules called ketones. When you get energy from carbohydrate-based foods, the carbohydrates are broken down into glucose.

Glucose, which is the simplest sugar molecule, is what provides the basic energy for our bodies. Every time you eat, the plant food you consume is broken down into glucose, which is then released into the bloodstream. It travels to the cells throughout the body, where it is used as an energy source for basic cellular functioning. Your brain, kidneys, and red blood cells are particularly dependent on glucose to derive the energy the cells need in order to stay alive and function properly. Think about the "brain fog" you will often feel if you have gone a long time without a meal and feel the need to eat.

While many cells in the body can get energy through fat via ketones, some cells in the brain, your red blood cells, and some cells in the kidneys require glucose to function. The brain must get about 30% of its energy needs from sugar. So even if you are not consuming much sugar in your diet, your body will maintain blood sugar above certain minimums.

Types of Sugars in the Diet

You derive glucose from the carbohydrates that you eat in your diet. This can include starches like potatoes, whole-grain breads and pastas, and fruits and vegetables. It also includes sugar, whether it's in the form of table sugar, desserts like candy and cake, fruit, or fruit juice.

Carbohydrates can be simple, or varying levels of complex. The simplest carbohydrate molecule is a single sugar, like glucose. Fructose is another example of a single sugar molecule. Table sugar, or sucrose, is actually a glucose molecule linked together with a fructose molecule. With just two molecules linked together, while it is a bit more complex and your body would break the bond during digestion, sucrose is still a very simple carbohydrate.

Carbohydrates can also belong to chains of glucose molecules linked together. These form starches and complex carbohydrates that take longer for the body to digest because it has to break all of the bonds in the molecule in order to liberate each of the glucose molecules in the chain so that they can be used for energy. This is done before releasing them to the bloodstream, where they contribute to the blood sugar.

If you eat a simple carbohydrate, your blood sugar will rise quickly, because the body doesn't have to spend any time breaking the molecules apart. If you eat a more complex carbohydrate, the body has to spend time breaking them apart, and so your blood sugar will rise more gradually. In either case, it is normal for your blood sugar to rise after a meal. But as we'll see, the way that it rises can be a strong indication that you are either healthy or having problems related to blood sugar and possibly diabetes.

There is another type of carbohydrate that humans cannot derive energy from. This is known as dietary fiber. When a food contains a significant amount of dietary fiber, it takes even longer to break the molecules apart into a form that can be digested. A complex carbohydrate can generally be assumed to have high levels of dietary fiber in it. Since the fiber has to be broken apart from the digestible components in the food, and then those have to be split apart into individual glucose molecules, it takes longer to digest foods that are complex carbohydrates, and they usually lead to a slower rise in blood sugar after digestion. As we will see, you can determine how complex the carbohydrates are in different food items and get some understanding of how they are digested by looking at the glycemic index of the food.

Metabolic Syndrome

Many of us in the modern world have a difficult time digesting carbohydrates. One of the ways that this will manifest in middle age is with the development of metabolic syndrome. This is a cluster of health measures that indicates the body is not handling blood sugar in a normal way.

A Fat Waistline

The first characteristic of metabolic syndrome is fat on the waistline. When this syndrome was first described, it was associated with the classic "beer belly" appearance in men. And that is not a surprise since beer contains many starches that can lead to problems if consumed in excess. Metabolic syndrome is definitely not linked to being male, of course. Middle-aged women can suffer from it as well – the key characteristic is abdominal fat that builds up over time. So if your waistline is expanding, you need to be keenly aware of metabolic syndrome.

Metabolic syndrome is not based on waistline alone, but rather you must have three or more of the characteristics associated with it. The second characteristic is an elevated fasting blood sugar. We will be talking in more detail about blood sugar levels in the next chapter, so don't be worried about the specifics right now. But if you have abnormally elevated blood sugar levels, this can be associated with metabolic syndrome.

High Blood Pressure

The next health marker associated with metabolic syndrome is elevated blood pressure. Although the exact causes are not precisely understood and can vary from individual to individual, weight gain often leads to higher blood pressure levels. If you have metabolic syndrome, you might have medically diagnosed high blood pressure, or you might just have "pre-hypertension" (high blood pressure is also called hypertension by medical professionals). High blood pressure is a serious health problem, and through the years, medical professionals have been changing the specific definitions because of the impacts that high blood pressure on health.

According to Harvard Medical School, the current definition of "normal" blood pressure is 120/80 or less. Pre-hypertension is taken to be 120-130 over 90 or less. If your blood pressure is above this level, it is considered "high blood pressure". Varying levels can indicate varying risks to health, and so it is divided into stages 1,2, and 3. Stage 1 high blood pressure is 130-139 over 80-90. Stage 2 high blood pressure is 140 and above 90 and above. If the upper number (called systolic) rises above 180, or the lower number (called diastolic) rises above 120, you are considered to have stage 3 high blood pressure, which is a very serious condition and possibly even an emergency.

It is important to understand high blood pressure because it is closely associated with high blood sugar and diabetes. There are many different reasons for this, one being the damage that high blood sugar can cause to blood vessels over time. High blood pressure is also associated with being overweight or obese, which is also associated with high blood sugar and diabetes. When you have a lot of excess body mass, your heart and blood vessels have to pump more blood and work harder to fuel all that extra weight. You may also retain more fluids if you are obese. These factors can lead to high blood pressure.

The tendency in the medical community is to treat high blood pressure with drugs, and due to the problems that can arise from high blood pressure, including heart attack and debilitating and potentially fatal strokes, this is necessary. However, if you have high blood pressure, you should be taking steps to reverse it through natural means, and get off the medications or reduce your dosages if possible. This will mean losing weight and engaging in regular exercise. You can also reduce blood pressure by consuming foods that contain natural nitrates like beets.

High Triglycerides

Another factor associated with metabolic syndrome is high triglycerides and low HDL cholesterol. Triglycerides are a type of fat that flows through the bloodstream. But although you might associate the idea of fat flowing through the bloodstream with the consumption of dietary fat, high triglycerides actually come from excess consumption of sugar. You can also get high triglycerides by consuming excess amounts of alcohol. In either case, the liver makes the triglycerides and releases them into the bloodstream. If you have high blood sugar, it won't be surprising if you also have high triglycerides – but that isn't going to happen in all cases. If you have high blood sugar but don't know your triglyceride level, you should ask your doctor to have it tested. Generally speaking a triglyceride level of 150 mg/dL or lower is considered healthy, and 100 mg/dL or lower is optimal. Any level above 150 mg/dL is unhealthy, and levels above 500 mg/dL can be dangerous.

High triglyceride levels can have many impacts on health. In fact, high triglycerides, and not high cholesterol levels, are more impactful on the development of heart disease. It has been demonstrated that a high triglyceride to HDL ratio is the best way to predict future heart attack risk when using blood markers to determine the state of health. It turns out that high triglyceride levels are associated with riskier cholesterol molecules.

You have probably learned at some point that there is "good" and "bad" cholesterol. Good cholesterol is known to scientists as HDL cholesterol, while bad cholesterol is known as LDL cholesterol. HDL cholesterol helps keep your blood vessels clean and open. LDL cholesterol can get stuck to your artery walls, leading over time to the formation of blockages and clots that can break off, causing heart attacks and stroke.

It turns out that the larger your LDL molecules, the less likely they are to cause problems in your arteries. But what we need to know right now is that high triglyceride levels are associated with smaller LDL molecules. That means that high triglycerides make it more likely that LDL molecules can stick to your artery walls leading to heart disease. In contrast, low triglyceride levels are associated with larger LDL molecules that don't get stuck, and so, in that case, you have a much lower risk of heart disease.

But here is another key takeaway that we already mentioned – remember that triglyceride levels are associated with carbohydrate consumption, in particular, simple carbohydrates. The more sugars you consume, and the higher your blood sugar, the higher your triglycerides are likely to be. Remember, this doesn't happen in all cases, but if you have high blood pressure you need to get this checked out.

There are three ways to lower triglyceride levels. The first is through medication. The most conventional medication is a drug called gemfibrozil, which was developed as an early cholesterol-lowering medication. It actually doesn't have much impact on cholesterol but turned out to be pretty effective at lowering triglycerides. However, it can have some unpleasant side effects, including slightly elevating the risk of developing appendicitis.

The second way to lower triglyceride levels is to consume large amounts of fish oil. This can be done either by eating large amounts of fatty fish or by consuming capsules or doing both. If you have elevated triglycerides, you are going to need to consume 3,000-4,000 mg per day of omega-3 fish oils in the form of EPA and DHA. Fish that are suitable for this purpose include mackerel, salmon, sardines, and anchovies among others. If you are using over the counter fish oils, you need to make sure that the dosages are appropriate – they need to contain the right levels of EPA and DHA. Eating fish is best, but many people have trouble eating enough fish, or they may not like the taste of fish at all.

You can also get a prescription fish oil from your doctor. This will ensure that you are getting the proper amount and quality of fish oil, in the right dosages. Check with your doctor about this if you have high triglycerides.

The last way to lower triglycerides is to eat a low carbohydrate diet. Remember that triglycerides are actually made by the liver out of sugar and/or alcohol consumed in the diet. By reducing the amounts of carbohydrates in your diet, you will reduce the amounts of triglycerides produced. Depending on the state of your health, you may have to severely restrict the amounts of carbohydrates consumed. However, you will find that since sugar and triglycerides are associated, this will simultaneously help reset your blood sugar to healthy levels.

Low HDL Cholesterol

As if high triglycerides were not bad enough, people with metabolic syndrome also tend to have low HDL cholesterol as well. Remember that HDL cholesterol helps to clean up your bloodstream. It will gather up excess LDL molecules and bring them back to the liver for processing. HDL can also help clean up the artery walls to inhibit the formation of blockages that lead to heart disease.

Your HDL level should be 40 mg/dL at a minimum. Ideally, it should be 50 mg/dL or higher. Low HDL levels are associated with an elevated risk of heart disease and stroke. At the present time, there is no medication that can effectively raise HDL levels, and there isn't a specific dietary change that can raise them either. However, losing weight can raise HDL levels.

Metabolic Syndrome and What it Means for You

You may have elevated blood sugars and have metabolic syndrome, or you may not. In any case, the development of metabolic syndrome is a serious warning sign for those that do develop it. If you have any of the health problems on this list, in particular at least three of them, and you also have elevated blood sugars, you need to start paying attention to your health now. Anyone who fails to take action on reversing metabolic syndrome is likely to develop type 2 diabetes, heart disease, increase their risk of stroke, and also increase their risk of cancer. If you are only now becoming aware that you have markers associated with metabolic syndrome, but your overall health is basically fine, you still have time to act. Even if you have become diabetic or developed other health problems associated with metabolic syndrome, changes to your diet and lifestyle can go a long way toward reversing it and restoring your body to health.

Side note: Fructose and Metabolic Syndrome

People have a mistaken belief that because fructose is associated with fruit, which is natural and generally healthy, that it's good for you. In fact, nothing could be further from the truth. First we need to distinguish between eating whole fruit, which is healthier because it has a lot of fiber, and so the digestion of any sugars in the fruit (which will include glucose, fructose, and sucrose) is going to be slowed by the fiber, and therefore your body is better able to handle it. Contrast this with fruit juice, where the fiber has been removed. Fruit juice consumption will cause your blood sugar to spike rapidly, and it's not good for you to consume even orange juice.

A recent study shows that damage that fruit juice consumption can cause. Scientists examined people drinking large amounts of orange juice, and they found that after just a month, they had high levels of triglycerides.

Consuming fructose appears to be even worse than glucose. Fructose, consumed in large amounts, can even cause liver damage and strain the pancreas. For some people, fructose consumption can be closely linked to the development of metabolic syndrome over time. At best, consumption of fruit juices, including orange juice should be done in moderation, and you might want to simply avoid it altogether.

The Role of Insulin

An important hormone is made by your pancreas that is important for the digestion of carbohydrates. This hormone is called insulin. It plays many roles in the body. The first and most important role of insulin is to get your cells to take up blood sugar out of the bloodstream so that they can use it to produce energy. When you are on the road to developing diabetes, your cells become insulin resistant. This means that they don't respond so well to the signals given by insulin to take up the blood sugar, and this is what leads to high blood sugar levels. Your body will respond by making more and more insulin over time.

This is not a good thing, as insulin has other effects on the body. One of these is that insulin tells the liver to burn excess blood sugar into fat and release it into the bloodstream. Then insulin signals your fat cells to take up that fat and store it. So now we see the connection between sugar and weight gain – first you begin having trouble taking up all the sugar, and then insulin gets that sugar made into fat and stored on the body.

People who are insulin resistant, which means people with high blood sugar and also people with metabolic syndrome, their insulin levels are chronically elevated.

Finally, insulin can cause the body to be in a state of stress, leading to higher levels of cortisol and other hormones. As a result, when insulin levels are chronically elevated, the body is in a constant state of biochemical stress. This can lead to inflammation and even increase your risk of cancer and other diseases.

Diabetes and Other Complications

Elevated blood sugars, left untreated, or not dealt with through natural means, will eventually lead to the development of diabetes. This is a condition whereby your blood sugars remain elevated and reach very high levels. Diabetes is a chronic condition, and many in the medical establishment believe it is permanent as well (we will see that it is neither chronic nor permanent). Left untreated, diabetes can cause many health problems.

Diabetes essentially results from insulin resistance. In the early stages, the pancreas is still able to make insulin, but it is unable to make enough to get your body to take up sugar properly. In the early stages, diabetes can be controlled by medications like metformin. This will help you maintain blood sugar levels in normal ranges. It will reduce the risks of complications and the development of secondary diseases related to high blood sugars. In fact, people taking metformin can reduce their risk of developing cancer by half.

However, in most patients, over time, the impact becomes less and less, and diabetes becomes more difficult to control. Eventually the pancreas will wear out and have a hard time producing insulin. This means that the patient will have to be given insulin as a medication through injections. At this point, you are full-blown diabetic and totally dependent on daily medications to even stay alive.

The problem with the standard medical approach is that it doesn't get to the core problem – which is insulin resistance. Instead of dealing with insulin resistance, patients are in a situation where they have to continually inject insulin, and many find they have to go with higher and higher doses as the years get by. Eventually, this results in worsening health.

Damage to Small Blood Vessels

Several serious complications can result from elevated blood sugar and insulin levels. The first is that high blood sugar levels damage the small blood vessels and capillaries throughout your body. This is really something basic, try imagining filling your blood vessels with honey or molasses. The sugar is going to clog up the smaller blood vessels, preventing blood from blowing properly. When blood is not flowing properly, your organs are going to get damaged.

Damage to Kidneys and High Blood Pressure

The kidneys are particularly susceptible to damage from this phenomenon. This is one reason that diabetics often have high blood pressure. The kidneys are intimately involved in the regulation of blood sugar, and they control the levels of various minerals like sodium and potassium in the blood, keeping them in the right balance to maintain healthy blood sugar levels. But if you become diabetic, the kidneys are going to get damaged from the high blood sugar and lose their ability to maintain healthy blood pressure levels. As a result, diabetics have elevated risk of stroke.

Blindness

Second, small capillaries are important for healthy eyes and vision. That means if you have chronically high blood sugars, you are going to get eye damage. If left untreated or not effectively dealt with, high blood sugar can eventually lead to blindness. Diabetes remains one of the leading causes of blindness.

Ulcerations and Amputation

High blood sugar also means that you are not going to be getting a good blood supply to your extremities, especially the feet and lower legs. This can lead to several complications. The first of these is you won't be getting adequate supplies of infection-fighting blood cells to these areas. If you get a cut on your foot, it can develop into a serious infection. People with untreated diabetes (and even some with treated diabetes) can develop severe, runaway infections as a result. This can result in the need for hospitalization, and in serious cases, amputation of feet or the lower legs.

Nerve Damage

Another aspect of diabetes and the complications that result from elevated blood sugar preventing normal blood flow is nerve damage. The degree of nerve damage can vary, but it can lead to feelings of tingling and numbness, in particular in the extremities of the hands and feet. This can worsen over time if blood sugar levels are not controlled.

Impotence

A condition related to nerve damage and problems with blood flow seen in diabetics is impotence in men.

Heart Disease and Stroke

Over time, the damage to blood vessels will increase. This can lead to the development of atherosclerosis or hardening of the arteries. Diabetics are at elevated risk of having a heart attack or stroke. In fact, a diabetic is twice or more likely than a person without diabetes to have a heart attack. This is true even when controlling for other factors like high cholesterol. Diabetics also have higher risk of having bad blood markers associated with heart disease including high cholesterol, high triglycerides, and low HDL cholesterol.

Cancer

Believe it or not, cancer is another "complication" of diabetes. Cancer cells strongly prefer, indeed, according to some researchers, need sugar in order to survive, grow, and develop into life-threatening tumors. As a result, the higher your blood sugar, the higher your risk of cancer. By the time you are diagnosed with diabetes, your risk of cancer can be double to quadruple that of the general population. One sign of this link is the fact that taking metformin appears to cut the risk of cancer in half. While that is heartening to consider, you are better off reducing your risk ahead of time using natural means of reducing blood sugar. So keep in mind the higher your fasting and average blood sugars, the higher your risk of developing cancer.

Dental Problems

Diabetics are also at higher risk of dental problems like gingivitis, tooth abscess, and cavities. This can lead to serious health consequences, including loss of your teeth, elevated heart disease risk, and serious infections, and even death. Once again, these problems result from inadequate blood supply through the small blood vessels and capillaries.

The Food Industry

Sadly, the food industry has helped to feed the diabetes epidemic over the past several decades. This goes back many years, even back to the early years of the 20th century. The food industry is focused on ease of production and profits. It turns out it's easier to make cheap foods that can be sold at a profit out of simple carbohydrates, and then consumers can be addicted to them by adding excess salt and sugar.

One area where this took off in the first half of the 20th century was with the invention of breakfast cereals made out of simple carbohydrates. This combined with the increased time pressure of Americans in the morning, as they had to eat something quick and be off to work and school.

Food manufacturers also opted to make cheap breads and other products using simple carbohydrates. That is, they used "white" processed flour to make white bread and other products while neglecting to make products out of whole grains. One result of this was people were consuming simple carbohydrates without the needed dietary fiber that would slow digestion, and help them to maintain better blood sugar levels.

After the second world war, the concept of "fast food" was invented, making the dietary problem even worse. Fast food focused on quick, cheap food that was loaded with simple carbohydrates, salt, and fat. People began leading even more rushed lives as the decades went by, and fast and processed foods became a larger part of their diets as a result. This eventually led to rising levels of obesity and diabetes.

Throughout the last decades of the 20th century, medical professionals began emphasizing low-fat diets. One result of this was people ate less fatty meats and oils and consumed ever-rising levels of carbohydrates and sugars.

The food industry has also pushed the consumption of sugary drinks. This has been going on for some time with the introduction of cokes and other sodas that contain large amounts of sugars, but it has also expanded to the availability of sugar-laden "energy" drinks, health drinks (supposedly healthy), and the marketing of fruit juices. The processed food industry also pushes the consumption of potato chips and other sugar or salt and fat-laden snacks.

The bottom line is that the food industry knows that certain combinations of carbohydrates, sugars, salt, and fat produce cheaply made but highly addictive foods. They have pushed these foods on the public without regard to the health impacts of processed foods. The best thing to do, of course, is to avoid consuming them except on occasion.

The Medical Establishment

Western medicine has been focused on treatment once you have a disease, and although it's now starting to change, hardly thinking about the prevention of diseases in the first place. One result of this is that the approach of conventional medical doctors to diabetes has been to focus on controlling the disease after the fact. Second, they have been focused on using pills, potions, and medications to control it. Once you are diagnosed with diabetes, you are going to be beholden to multiple pharmaceuticals for life, and you will create an endless stream of money into the medical establishment.

This is not to say that individual doctors don't believe that they are helping patients. They certainly do, but like many of us, they have been brainwashed into thinking that fixing something with a pill is the only way to approach things.

The underlying belief, when it comes to blood sugar and diabetes, is that the condition will only get worse over time, and it cannot be reversed. According to the conventional medical establishment, diabetes is chronic and progressive. All that can be done is to manage it with the right pills or insulin injections. Then you also have to try and manage the inevitable complications that will arise as a result.

Many patients don't think about it because insurance pays a lot of the bills. But you are generating thousands of dollars for the medical establishment once you are hooked on these medications, and they will only slow the progress of the disease, not cure it.

Recently I read of a diabetes doctor that went to a conference on dietary habits and diabetes. He noted with a large sense of irony, the fact that the attendees of the conference were fed a meal heavy on carbohydrates and sugars. In fact, many large associations like the American Diabetes Association advocate for diets that actually encourage the development and progression of diabetes, rather than reverse it. It is almost as though the medical establishment is hoping to encourage people to develop the disease.

After all, a large number of people with a chronic disease creates a situation where millions of people are going to be buying large quantities of medications for the rest of their lives in order to "manage" their conditions. The insurance companies will profit as well since they are often the ones getting higher premiums from the public to help pay for all these medications. Of course ironically, if you develop diabetes you will be labeled as having a "pre-existing condition" and you might be denied insurance coverage.

This is not to say that you should not take your metformin or insulin if it has been prescribed. You should definitely follow the advice of your doctor, and if you are already on these medications, getting off of them is going to take some care, but it can be done. There are natural ways to control blood sugar and even cure diabetes. Weight loss is very important in helping with this, along with changes to dietary and exercise habits.

However, you should find a doctor that is friendly toward more natural approaches. That way, they can properly help you head in the right direction with lifestyle changes while managing your medications along the way and helping you to get off of the medications at the right time. For those that are not yet diabetic, you can save a fortune in future insurance premiums and copayments including for medications by dealing with your blood sugar problems now, in a natural way.

Weight loss, exercise, and other lifestyle changes can help you keep your blood sugar under control, and help you to avoid developing diabetes and all of the health complications that are associated with it. In the rest of this book, we hope to help set you on the right path to healing your blood sugar naturally.

In the next chapter, we are going to talk about blood sugar in a more detailed way. We will learn what levels of blood sugar are considered healthy and how blood sugar changes when we eat and sleep, or throughout the day. We will also discuss the ways that aging can impact blood sugar, and we'll also talk about the relationship between blood sugar and pregnancy. Understanding what normal blood sugar levels are will help you to get better control of your health.

Chapter 2: Blood Sugar Levels

Knowledge is power, and taking control of your health when it comes to blood sugar levels starts with understanding what normal blood sugar levels are. In the last chapter, we mentioned many of the health problems and complications that can result from chronically elevated blood sugar levels, but if you don't know what normal blood sugar levels are and how they should vary, there is no way to know what the true state of your health is. We hope to clear that up in this chapter and give you the information that you need in order to take control of your health. Knowing what healthy levels of blood sugar are is the first step to having an awareness of where your health is and helping you to know when you are heading in the right direction.

Spikes vs. Long Term Elevations

It is important to note both spikes in blood sugar and long-term elevations of blood sugar. Both can be damaging to your health. One of the problems with blood sugar spikes is many people who have them aren't aware of it, even if they are monitoring their own blood sugar. This can happen when you focus on your fasting blood sugar levels. While fasting blood sugar levels are important, and they are a major indicator of the status of your health, blood sugar levels after consuming food are important as well.

Spikes occur when blood sugar rises to a very high level over a shorter time period. If you have constant spikes in blood sugar, then you might be experiencing damage to your blood vessels. For this reason being aware of blood sugar spikes is an important part of your overall attention to blood sugar health.

Normal Blood Sugar

By the time you read this, the definitions of what normal blood sugar is may have changed a little. As it is with high blood pressure, elevated blood sugars are a serious problem, and this has led to pressure in the medical establishment to create more strict definitions of what healthy blood sugar is. However, there can be a bit of zealotry with this that isn't very realistic. For this reason, I am going to stick to the traditional definitions of normal blood sugar levels, which are more reasonable for determining the state of your health and also which are more reasonable for considering blood sugar in the context of an aging population.

Fasting Blood Sugar

The first blood sugar number that you need to be aware of is your fasting blood sugar level. This is the blood sugar level after going 8-12 hours without consuming any food. You can consume water, but you should avoid all food items before getting tested for a fasting blood sugar level.

The fasting blood sugar level is the most fundamental number that is used in determining how healthy your blood sugar is. It not only gives you a baseline of your blood sugar levels, it also tells us something about the state of your liver health and the role it is playing in your blood sugar level. The reason for this is that the liver actually makes sugar out of the food you eat, and it will also store sugar. When you are not consuming food, your liver is going to be releasing sugar into the blood, even during fasting periods.

The reason that the liver releases sugar into the blood while you are fasting is that the body must maintain a narrow range of blood sugar levels in order to survive. In the first chapter we mentioned that the brain must get 30% of its energy from sugar in order to remain operational. The other 70% of the brain will get its energy from sugar as well when blood sugar levels are elevated, but it can also get its energy from fat in the form of ketones. Red blood cells, which carry oxygen to the various parts and organs of the body, must have sugar in order to survive. There are also certain cells in the kidneys that must have sugar, and so for these reasons your body must keep blood sugar from going below a certain minimum.

Normal fasting blood sugar levels range from a low of 70 mg/dL up to 110 mg/dL. Some doctors are becoming more strict, and define this range to be 70-100 mg/dL, but staying with the 110 mg/dL upper limit is more reasonable.

Low Blood Sugar

If your blood sugar is too low, this is a condition referred to as hypoglycemia. If it gets too low, low blood sugar can become a very serious medical problem. Any value less than 70 mg/dL is considered hypoglycemic, but the cutoff of 54 mg/dL or lower is considered a medical emergency. If at any time, you find that your blood sugar drops below 70 mg/dL, you should consume some carbohydrates in order to raise it back to within the normal range.

Although it's ironic because diabetes is a disease of high blood sugars, low blood sugar is a constant risk factor in the life of a diabetic. For this reason, many diabetics keep a supply of glucose tablets on hand for emergencies. By consuming blood sugar tablets, you can instantly raise your blood sugar because there isn't any digestion necessary, and as soon as it passes through your stomach and into the small intestine the glucose in the tablets can start to be released into the bloodstream and restore blood sugar levels to normal values.

Failure to deal with extremely low blood sugar levels can cause major medical problems, and it can even be fatal. One problem that can result from hypoglycemia is coma. Remember that your brain needs a constant supply of fuel, and if it isn't able to get that fuel, it will start to shut down. Coma can result, and in some cases, the patient may not recover and could end up dying.

Prediabetic Fasting Glucose Levels

If your fasting blood sugar is at least 110 mg/dL but less than 125 mg/dL, you are said to be pre-diabetic. This means that you are prone to developing diabetes, probably headed towards developing diabetes, but you are not quite there yet. If you are prediabetic, you should actually thank your lucky stars. Why?

If you are prediabetic, that means that lifestyle changes are likely to be effective at reversing the condition. Someone who is prediabetic but continues with the same lifestyle, especially if that is leading to weight gain, is likely to become a full-blown diabetic. When that happens, you are probably going to be put on one or more medications, and you might even be put on insulin. When these things happen, while it's not impossible, it can become far more difficult to reverse the situation using natural means, and more drastic measures may be necessary.

When you are prediabetic, most doctors are not going to put you on medication, and those that are inclined to put you on medication (probably low dose metformin) are going to be open to changes in diet and lifestyle, including exercise. You may have to be assertive when dealing with your doctor, but if they are convinced that you will make the needed changes, they are probably going to allow you to have several months to do so.

Keep in mind that when you are prediabetic, damage is already being done to your body. While you might not be at the point of having kidney and eye damage or be developing high levels of heart disease, you are already on that path once your blood sugars have become elevated. Any blood sugar level that above 110 mg/dL after fasting should be taken very seriously.

Diabetes and Fasting Blood Glucose Levels

Any fasting blood sugar level of 125 mg/dL and above can be an indication of diabetes. In this case, a single test result is not going to be enough for a diagnosis. We will talk about diagnosis in the next chapter, but for now, keep the number in mind and note that at the very least, they are going to want to confirm with a second test result and also do some other tests. If your fasting blood sugar level has gone higher than 130 mg/dL, you are definitely in the diabetic range.

Eating and Blood Sugar Levels

Of course, eating a meal that contains any level of carbohydrates is going to raise your blood sugar. The time it takes to raise it is going to range between 1-2 hours. We will talk about testing your blood sugar after eating in the next chapter, but a typical peak that a normal person is going to see after consuming a standard meal is 140 mg/dL. If you find that you have higher peak blood sugar levels after meals, this is a major red flag. The higher the peak is, the more dangerous it is. Remember that blood sugar spikes can damage the small blood vessels throughout your body. The higher the peak and the longer it lasts, the more damage that is going to be done.

So for "normal' levels, 140 mg/dL or lower after consuming a meal is the target.

Variation of Blood Sugar Levels

We have already touched on two major variations of blood sugar levels. One is after fasting, which helps to establish your baseline blood sugar level while also giving us an idea of how much sugar your liver is making and releasing into the bloodstream. It also tells us the state of your body with respect to insulin; if you have a higher fasting blood sugar level, this tells us that the cells are not being so responsive to insulin which is trying to get them to take up that blood sugar and use it for energy production. Other things can impact blood sugar levels.

Sleep and Blood Sugar Levels

Sleep can have a major impact on blood sugar levels. Let's begin by considering what your blood sugar levels should be when going to bed. The generally accepted range is 90-150 mg/dL. The higher end of the range is used for diabetics. Keep in mind the second role that insulin plays in the body, which is to direct sugar, which is leftover or in excess into body fat. This is one of the reasons that eating right before bedtime or in the middle of the night can lead to weight gain. If you consume food under those conditions, when you go to bed afterward, your body is not going to be as physically active and so won't need the sugar. That means that it's going to be put away and stored as body fat.

For a person who is not diabetic, you would want to be going to bed with a blood sugar that is around 90-110 mg/dL. Diabetics are allowed to have a higher range.

When you sleep, as blood sugar levels naturally drop, the liver is going to be releasing sugar into the bloodstream in order to keep blood sugar levels at a healthy level, so that the brain, red blood cells, and kidneys, along with other systems and organs of the body, get the minimal amount of sugar they need in order to keep functioning properly.

It's interesting to note that sleep plays an important role in maintaining healthy blood sugar levels, however. People who get a good nights' sleep of 7-8 hours, on average, tend to have healthier blood sugar levels. While lack of sleep is not a cause of diabetes, it can contribute to unhealthy blood sugar levels.

Scientists have found that sleeping for shorter periods each night changes the amounts and types of hormones flowing throughout the body. One impact of this is that the less sleep you get, the less glucose tolerance you have. That means you are likely to end up with high blood sugar levels over time if this becomes a habit. When you are sleep deprived, the body has less deep sleep, a period of time during the night when cortisol levels decrease, and the brain reduces its need for sugar. Reduction in the level of cortisol and the background levels of insulin during deep sleep can help the body control body fat and weight gain. In fact, although there are many different factors that can impact a person's weight, it has been shown that sleep deprivation can help to contribute to long-term weight gain. Weight gain by itself is connected to higher blood sugar levels, and so this, in turn, helps drive elevated blood glucose.

Variation of Blood Sugar Throughout the Day

When you wake up in the morning, you can think of your blood sugar level as being at the "baseline." From here, it is going to go up and down depending on your consumption of food and the activity that you engage in. Exercise is going to play a role in decreasing blood sugar levels.

However, blood sugar levels will also undergo a natural cycle of rising and falling in response to the food that you eat.

So if you eat three meals per day, you are going to see your blood sugar rise three times a day to a peak level that should be 140 mg/dL or less. The ideal and most health level is actually about 125 mg/dL. In any case, if you are not diabetic, you will see your blood sugar gradually rise to the peak value, and then reduce back to the baseline. The time required to do this will be about 2-3 hours, with a peak coming maybe one or possibly two hours after eating.

As the day wears on, you will have your blood sugar stabilize near fasting blood sugar levels when you go to bed, assuming that this has been 2-4 hours after your last meal. Then your blood sugar levels are going to rise slightly before you wake up the following morning. In part, your blood sugar levels will rise a little bit in order to give your brain enough fuel to wake up and begin the day.

Someone who is prediabetic is going to experience a different set of circumstances throughout the day with their blood sugar levels. In the early morning hours, the blood sugar level may be about the same as a healthy person. It might be slightly higher, ranging around 110-120 mg/dL. It could even be toward the healthy range of around 100-105 mg/dL, but the condition of prediabetes would be revealed when monitoring changes throughout the entire day. A prediabetic (or a diabetic in the early or more moderate stages) will see big differences while consuming food and in the aftermath.

First off, you are going to see a much sharper rise in your blood sugar, and it will reach a higher peak value. When you are either prediabetic or in the early stages of diabetes, your blood sugar might be peaking at 180-200 mg/dL after eating a meal that contains significant amounts of carbohydrate.

But that's not all. It will take longer for your blood sugar to decline, and it might not even drop back down to background levels, and instead, it could linger, remaining around 115 mg/dL to 125 mg/dL all the way to your next meal. So someone who is prediabetic or in the early stages of diabetes could be experiencing long periods of time throughout the day where their blood sugar remains elevated to one degree or another, causing constant damage to the blood vessels and the organs of the body.

This situation can continue until dinner when the unfortunate patient will experience another high blood sugar peak, followed by a gradual but prolonged drop off of blood sugar levels. While it might take a normal person just 2-3 hours to see their blood sugar drop back to normal, background levels, a prediabetic or early-stage diabetic might have to wait 5-6 hours before they see their blood sugar drop back to fasting levels or close to it. That long delay is why the prediabetic may experience elevated blood sugars, even if they are not dramatic, all day long. The only time blood sugar levels will drop back down to normal ranges or at least reasonably close to it, is during sleep.

As you might imagine, those chronically elevated levels of blood sugar can cause many health problems, including leading to heart and kidney disease. High blood sugars like that which last throughout the day can also feed cancer cells, leading to the development of clinical disease.

A diabetic who is "treated" using the standard methods preferred by the medical establishment might see similar patterns in their blood sugar throughout the day.

For a full-blown diabetic, who is not treated and who has had the condition for some time, the situation is even worse. To begin with, an untreated diabetic is going to have high fasting blood sugar levels. This can be in the range of 135 mg/dL all the way up to around 175 mg/dL. So even during sleep, the full-blown diabetic's body is dealing with high blood sugar levels and all the health complications that result from that.

When the untreated diabetic eats a meal containing any significant level of carbohydrate, the blood sugar will rise to dramatic peaks. Depending on the severity of the condition and how long they have had it without receiving treatment, blood sugar values can peak at 280-325 mg/dL after a meal, or even more in some cases. It will take hours for blood sugar levels to drop, but they are not going to drop nearly enough. They could drop to levels of maybe 200 mg/dL, but then it will be time to eat again, and so they will experience another rise in blood sugar levels to 300 mg/dL or more. This process will continue through the last meal, and then going to bed, the blood sugar will drop a bit, back down to whatever the fasting level is, and a little bit lower. Once again, blood sugar levels will rise a bit as the time to wake up arrives.

So for the diabetic, the problems of constantly elevated blood sugar are even worse. This means more damage to the systems of the body, and feeding the cancer cells all the sugar that they need to grow and thrive if any are present – obviously not something that you want happening inside your body.

All that Blood Sugar – and No Energy

Ironically, even though a diabetic has such high blood sugar levels, they are likely to feel tired and fatigued. The reason is simple – the sugar that provides the energy is flowing around in the blood, but not much of it is going into the cells where it's needed for energy. As a result, diabetics will feel tired throughout the day. This can have an impact on you no matter how mild your elevated blood sugar is or if you have undiagnosed or untreated full-blown diabetes.

Exercise and Blood Sugar

Exercise can lower blood sugar as well as sleep can. The amount of reduction in blood sugar levels is going to depend on the type, duration, and intensity of the exercise. The muscles themselves store blood sugar in the form of a starch called glycogen, which is also stored in the liver. When you exercise, the muscles are going to utilize it in order to have energy to do work. Any glycogen used during exercise must be replenished, which can help to lower blood sugar.

If you engage in long-lasting aerobic activity, which means 30 minutes per session or more, you will be using a lot of blood sugar, and this can help to maintain normal blood sugar levels. It has been shown that blood sugar levels will be reduced for 24 hours or more from an intense session of exercise that lasts long enough. Although full-blown diabetics won't be able to lower their blood sugar all the way down to normal levels, they can still benefit from this effect.

The more frequently you exercise, the more continuous this effect will be, and the more health benefits you will get from exercising in helping you to maintain healthy blood sugar levels, among other effects. In addition to help using up sugar currently in the blood, using your large muscles will help make them more efficient at taking sugar out of the blood and using it. This means that exercise can help to reduce insulin resistance and improve glucose tolerance.

For these reasons, anyone worried about high blood sugar should work to get more exercise into their daily routine. It will help improve your overall health while also helping you to reach your blood sugar goals.

Variation of Blood Sugar with Age

Does blood sugar naturally increase with age? It is generally accepted that the body doesn't work as well as we age, and so you might be inclined to think that some worsening blood sugar levels with age is something that is normal. To a certain extent, that might be true, but studies have shown that with the right diet and exercise habits, it is possible to maintain healthy blood sugar levels well into your 60s and 70s. In fact, maintaining healthy blood sugar levels can be an important component in avoiding the development of dementia. Although the brain certainly needs glucose, studies have actually shown that high blood glucose levels can cause brain damage. The effects are subtle, and so they occur over the course of decades and might not be apparent until much later in life.

Many scientists now believe that controlling blood sugar levels through diet, exercise, and, if necessary, through pharmaceutical interventions can help reduce the incidence and severity of dementia and generalized cognitive decline. It is not known what the association with severe cases of dementia like Alzheimer's is, but reducing supposedly normal cognitive decline is one area where controlling blood sugar can have a definite impact. In addition, although a definite cause and effect has not been established, the development of diabetes is associated with a higher risk of Alzheimer's.

Blood Sugar During Pregnancy

Many women are familiar with a health problem that is called gestational diabetes. During pregnancy, problems maintaining healthy blood sugar levels can develop. A distinction should be made between women who are already diabetic and who get pregnant and those who are not diabetic before pregnancy but develop gestational diabetes. One reason that diabetes and pregnancy is an important issue is that elevated blood sugar levels in the mother will have an impact on the developing baby as well.

Most doctors recommend that women get screened for gestational diabetes at about 24 weeks into the pregnancy. Depending on the results, doctors may recommend dietary changes, possibly exercise, and maybe even prescription medications to keep blood sugar within healthy ranges. It is not recommended that women who are pregnant try losing weight. If you know you are going to be pregnant at some point in the future, it is recommended that you get to a healthy weight before pregnancy, if possible.

High blood sugar levels by themselves during pregnancy don't necessarily mean that you have gestational diabetes. A doctor will likely do follow up tests, including a glucose tolerance test (see next chapter), to determine if diabetes is really present.

In most cases, gestational diabetes will resolve after childbirth. However, your doctor will probably do repeated tests to make sure you are returning to normal, assuming that you did not have any symptoms of diabetes before pregnancy.

Gestational diabetes can have many long-lasting impacts on the developing baby. The first of these is high birth weight, but the most important thing is that it can give the baby an elevated risk of developing type 2 diabetes in adulthood. Early birth can also result, and the baby may be born hypoglycemic.

Gestational diabetes is also associated with dangerously high blood pressure in the mother, which could lead to serious health complications.

For these reasons, it is recommended that you get tested and take appropriate steps to deal with any blood sugar problems during pregnancy.

Chapter 3: Diagnosis

Now you have some understanding of what normal blood sugars are; we can talk about diagnosis. One high blood sugar reading is not going to be enough to diagnose diabetes. If you show up with a high blood sugar reading, your doctor is going to want to investigate further in order to determine whether or not diabetes is really present. Depending on where you fall in the spectrum, your doctor may prescribe dietary and lifestyle changes, oral medications, or injectable insulin. In this chapter we are going to learn what specific tests are used and which tests you can do at home.

7 Signs of High Blood Sugar (even without diabetes)

Before we get into testing, we are going to look at some signs of high blood sugar that can occur with or without diabetes. In many cases, you can have mildly elevated blood sugars without even knowing it, but the more elevated your blood sugar becomes, the more likely it is you are going to start showing symptoms. In this section we are going to look at the seven most common symptoms that are encountered by people with high blood sugar. Keep in mind that since you may not show symptoms at all, it is important to get tested at least once a year by your doctor. If you have a family history of diabetes, you should consider getting a home test kit to check your blood sugar yourself on a periodic basis. We will talk about measuring blood glucose levels in later sections, but let's look at the top seven signs you might have diabetes or high blood sugar first.

Frequent Urination

The first sign that many people encounter when they have high blood sugar is a need to go to the bathroom frequently. They might find that they also have to get up in the middle of the night to urinate. The reason for this symptom, which may be subtle at first, is that the body is trying to get rid of the excess blood sugar. In fact, you can actually test for blood sugar in the urine. The body recognizes that blood sugar levels are high, and so the kidneys try to get rid of some of it by making you urinate more frequently.

Feeling Thirsty All The Time

This symptom is a direct result of the first symptom. Obviously, if you are urinating a lot more, you are going to get thirsty. You are going to need to drink a lot of water in order to replace what was lost. Again, in the early stages of high blood sugar, this symptom might be somewhat subtle. But you might also find that as time goes on, it gets harder and harder to quench your thirst. You might find that your throat and mouth often feel dry and that you can't seem to get rid of this situation, and you're never quite satisfied.

Chronic Hunger

When you are suffering from diabetes, or just high blood sugar generally, your body is not able to utilize the blood sugar that is flowing around in your body. As a result, the cells in your body are going to be suffering from energy fatigue. One consequence of this is that you are going to be feeling hungry all the time. You might eat a meal of carbohydrates, and even if it is a significant quantity of food, you'll discover that it doesn't quite satisfy.

Nerve Pain or Tingling

If you have been suffering from high blood sugar for a prolonged period, you might experience a lot of tingling sensations. You might also experience some level of nerve pain, especially in the extremities of your fingers and toes. The reason that this happens is when you have chronically elevated blood sugars; your nerve endings are not going to be getting an adequate blood supply. They are supplied by small blood vessels and capillaries, and as we mentioned earlier, these tiny blood vessels can literally get stuck up with sugar. When that happens, your nerve endings can be damaged, leading to these sensations. You might feel the sensation of prickly needles in your hands and feet, or it might seem like various parts of your body are "going to sleep" all the time. Of course, there can be other causes of these sensations, some harmless. So it's important to confirm by actually finding out what your blood sugar levels actually are.

Dark Skin Patches

One interesting symptom that prediabetics and undiagnosed diabetics get is darkened patches of skin. This is actually caused by elevated insulin levels. Remember that when you are developing diabetes, your cells get resistant to insulin. That is, for a given amount of insulin, they stop responding as the insulin tries to get them to take up glucose out of the blood. The body reacts to this situation by continually releasing more and more insulin. This can damage the skin leading to dark patches. The most common locations for these dark patches are in the groin area, the armpits, and the neck. The skin can also become thickened in these areas.

Skin Tags

Everyone is probably going to get some skin tags as they age, but if you are developing a lot of skin tags, in particular in the armpits and neck area, high blood sugars might be the culprit. This is related to the dark skin patches discussed above; it is from damage to the skin caused by high levels of circulating insulin. Again, this is something that you want to confirm by finding out what your blood sugars actually are. Don't assume that because you have some skin tags that you have high blood sugars.

Slow Healing Wounds

As we have discussed before, when you have high blood sugars, you are getting less blood supply to extremities of the body like your lower legs and feet. This means that these areas of the body are not getting enough oxygen, nutrients carried by the blood, and white blood cells that are necessary to fight infection. As a result, if you get a wound, it may take longer than normal to heal. This is a complication that is likely to result later on in the process, and so if you are at the early stages of dealing with high blood pressure, you might not have this symptom. As the condition progresses, it can get worse. In people with higher blood sugars, particularly those who are in the diabetic range but untreated, a wound can result in a severe infection that could even lead to the necessity of amputation of a finger, toe, or even afoot.

Bonus: More Signs of High Blood Sugar

There are actually more than seven signs you have high blood sugar. Chronic fatigue can be a sign that you are having blood sugar issues. Fatigue results because the cells of your body are not getting the adequate supply of energy they need to function normally.

Another sign is feeling hungry soon after eating. This can be an early sign that your body is not handling and metabolizing carbohydrate-based foods properly. If this describes your situation, it could be an indication that you could nip your problem in the bud by following a low carbohydrate diet.

Blurry vision is a sign of high blood sugar when it has gone untreated for a long-time period, and it's progressing through full-blown diabetes. This can happen from a blood sugar spike after a meal, and the blood sugar entering the small blood vessels of the eye can cause visual disturbances, since the cells and components of the eye may be getting inadequate blood supply. Blurry vision will resolve when blood sugar levels drop back down, but if left untreated this will eventually lead to blindness.

Finally, unexplained weight loss can be a symptom of high blood sugar levels. Unfortunately, this is a sign that shows up late in the process. Normally, losing weight (when intentional) is something that can lessen the severity of diabetes and even reverse it and eliminate high blood sugar problems. But if you are experiencing unexplained weight loss as a symptom of high blood sugar levels, you are probably suffering from an advanced stage of the disease, and it might not be possible for you to manage it without medication, at least at first. Hopefully our readers have not yet reached this state – and you can do something about your blood sugar before you do. But if you are in this condition, see a doctor immediately. Unexplained weight loss accompanied by the other signs discussed in this section can be a definite indicator that you have high blood sugars and possibly even diabetes. Unexplained weight loss can also be a sign of other serious diseases and conditions such as cancer.

How to Test Blood Sugar

There are several different ways that blood sugar can be tested. Some of these methods can be used at home, and this even includes some of the more important and advanced methods of blood glucose testing.

Fasting Plasma Test

The go-to test for monitoring blood sugar levels is called the fasting glucose test or fasting plasma test. This is to establish a baseline of what your blood sugar is when awakening in the morning. Remember that throughout the day, this sets a baseline level, and your blood sugar is going to be at this level or higher throughout the day. You should fast between 8-12 hours before taking this test.

A fasting glucose test is going to be a standard testing method that is done by your doctor after your annual exam. The test, by itself, is not definitive. For one thing, you can have a normal fasting glucose level but have spikes that are high and long-lasting, leading to a higher average blood sugar that can be problematic. Alternatively, you might have a one-time result that is not really indicative of your typical fasting blood sugar. For that reason, if you show up with a high fasting blood sugar, your doctor might want to repeat the test or perform other tests to confirm or reject what was seen from that one particular result.

If you have not had problems with blood sugar before, you should have a fasting blood glucose test at least once a year. Those who have a family history of diabetes might want to keep a closer tab on their blood sugar levels and do additional testing at home. We will discuss that in more detail in the next section.

Oral Glucose Tolerance Test

Remember that we discussed the different ways that healthy and unhealthy people will respond to the ingestion of a meal. If you are having problems with high blood sugar, your blood sugar might start from a normal or elevated baseline and spike quite high. It might take a long time to drop if your body is suffering from insulin resistance, which makes it difficult for the cells to take up sugar out of the blood.

bloodstream is something that can be tested in a doctor's office. They will have you ingest some sugar, usually in the form of a sugary drink. Then they will test your blood sugar at various intervals in order to get a clear picture of how your body responds to the ingestion of carbohydrates. This will include determining whether or not your blood sugar reaches a normal peak value, and how rapidly it declines after doing so. If your blood sugar rises to a high peak value and takes a long time to decline to normal levels, and you have shown other signs like a high fasting glucose level, you may receive a diagnosis of diabetes.

A1C Test

The A1C test is one of the most important tests that you can take to determine whether or not you are suffering from high blood sugar. In short, the A1C test will determine the average of your blood sugar over the past 90 days. It is sometimes referred to as the hemoglobin test because glucose molecules bind to hemoglobin in the blood, which is a part of the red blood cell that carries oxygen. If you have high blood sugar, more glucose molecules are going to be attached to your hemoglobin molecules. The reason that it is able to give you the average blood glucose over 90 days is the fact that red blood cells live, on average, about three months.

The results of the test are given as a percentage, so it will tell you what percent of hemoglobin had glucose molecules attached to them. The higher your blood sugar was, on average over the past 90 days, the higher the percentage is going to be. This can give a doctor a true picture of your blood sugar. Many patients will have a normal fasting glucoseose level, but they will be experiencing spikes in blood sugar after eating. That is something that does not show up on a fasting glucose test, or any standard glucose test because those types of tests only measure your blood glucose level at one instant of time.

It is important to know what the normal ranges are for the A1C test. The standard cutoff point between normal and problematic is 5.7%. So if you have an A1C test result of 5.7% or lower, you are considered to have normal blood sugar. If your fasting blood sugar is also normal, you will be considered to be in a healthy state as far as blood sugar is concerned.

The range for prediabetes is considered to be 5.7% up to 6.4%. If your A1C test falls in this range, you are at high risk of developing diabetes, but your doctor will probably advise changes in dietary and lifestyle habits in addition to losing weight if you are also overweight or obese.

If you have an A1C test result of 6.5% or higher, this is a strong indication of diabetes. Keep in mind that we are talking about type 2 diabetes here, more on that in the next chapter. Generally speaking, the higher the number is, the worse off your condition is. So if you are in the prediabetic range, a value of 5.8% might not be too concerning, but a value of 6.3% is a case where major intervention is going to become necessary in order to avoid becoming diabetic.

The A1C test may be used to test a woman during pregnancy, but it is not generally used to test for gestational diabetes. Rather, it would be used to establish whether or not a woman was showing signs of diabetes before pregnancy, and so would be performed early in the pregnancy to get an average blood sugar for the three months prior. An oral glucose test could be used in conjunction with routine blood tests to determine whether gestational diabetes has developed at 24 weeks or so into the pregnancy.

Random Check

A random check of blood glucose can be done using an ordinary blood plasma test in order to determine if your blood sugar is in normal ranges, given the circumstances. In particular you will want to note if the blood sugar goes above 180 mg/dL or worse above 200 mg/dL, and if it does how long it has been since eating and what was consumed. Random tests can be used to help establish a baseline.

How to Use a Glucometer

Testing your blood glucose at home is very easy. You can get ordinary glucometers that can be used to do a fasting blood glucose test or to test at various intervals, or engage in random testing. It is important to avoid cutting corners when getting a glucometer. My recommendation is to get on Amazon and read reviews of people who have already purchased and used various models. This will help you to determine the most accurate devices that you can fit in with your budget. Given the seriousness of getting accurate results, if you are tempted to simply go with the cheapest model you can find, I would urge you to avoid falling into that temptation.

In order to use the glucometer, you are going to need some lancelets to draw blood, alcohol swabs so that you don't end up getting an infection from poking yourself, and the appropriate test strips. I also advise getting a notebook in order to record your results, even though many monitors will keep tabs of your most recent readings.

Start by noting the date and time and the circumstances of the reading. For example, are you taking the reading after fasting 8 hours? Or are you taking the reading an hour after eating? These details need to be recorded.

Begin by washing your hands and then drying them. Believe it or not, having contaminants on your hand can cause erroneous readings. This can include having handled something sugary. So don't eat a donut and then go test your blood sugar without thoroughly washing and drying your hands first.

Next, insert the test strip into your device. Most modern glucometers will turn on automatically after you insert the test strip. Shake your hands a little bit in order to get an appropriate level of blood into your fingers. You can also rub them to warm them up, which will help increase the blood flow.

Then wipe your finger that you are going to use with an alcohol swab, and then poke it with the lancelet to draw blood. Always use a fresh needle or lancelet, never reuse items used to draw blood. Then put the blood drop on your test strip. Most glucometers only require a very small amount of blood in order to get a reading.

Then note the reading. If it is unusual or unexpected, you might want to duplicate the reading. When testing at home with a small amount of blood, errors can occur.

Mistakes in Testing

It's possible to make mistakes while testing. The first and most common mistake is not getting enough blood. Make sure that you can get a solid blood drop on your finger to put on the test strip. Squeeze your finger if necessary to get some more blood out. If you have an inadequate amount of blood, the reading on the meter might not be trustworthy.

The second mistake, as noted above, is having contaminants on your hand. In addition to the importance of sanitation, that is not wanting to inject bad bacteria into your bloodstream when you poke your finger; you want to make sure that something that could lead to an erroneous result is not on your hands. This can include sugar that you have touched from any substance that contains sugar, such as desserts, candy, or fruit juice. The blood glucometer will just measure the sugar; it can't tell where it originally came from if you are not following proper procedures. Washing and drying your hands thoroughly (with a clean towel) can ensure that you are not contaminating the reading.

Another common mistake that can occur is failing to fast long enough. If you are going to try and get a fasting reading at home, it is important to make sure that you have fasted for at least eight hours, and up to twelve is preferable. Sometimes people get up in the middle of the night and eat something and then take a "fasting" blood glucose test. The fact that you ate is going to skew the results and make your blood sugar look worse than it actually is.

Another surprising mistake made by many people is being in a state of dehydration when having a test done or doing a test at home. Blood sugar is reported as a density, and so if you have less water in your system – and therefore less water in your blood – you are going to end up with the result that could be erroneously high. Make sure that you are getting enough water to drink, and the night before a fasting glucose test do your best to stay hydrated. It can also help to get more accurate results by drinking a large glass of water an hour or two before your test.

Also, once you've washed your hands, avoid touching your face or mouth, or other objects with the finger you are going to use for testing. Just like getting sugar on your finger before doing the test and not washing it off can lead to erroneous results, touching your face or an object with your finger after you've washed your hands can also lead to contamination.

Failing to properly calibrate your meter can also result in erroneous readings. Most blood sugar meters are going to come with a test solution. People being what they are, can get anxious about going forward with a test and won't bother to use the test solution. The details vary depending on the meter, so we can't give specific instructions here, but you should read the manual that comes with your meter and use the test solution to do the calibration. This will give you some assurance that the meter is, in fact, working correctly. Typically, they will tell you what the reading should be from the solution so that you can know whether or not the machine is calibrated properly. If it isn't, follow the instructions that come with your meter.

Finally, it can be tempting to find out what your blood sugar level is after consuming a meal. One mistake that is commonly made is people test too soon after a meal. Please refer to the next section for the best times to test.

Monitoring Blood Sugar Levels at Home

When you are taking fasting glucose levels at home, if you are not yet diabetic but worried about high blood sugars, it is not necessary to take your blood sugar on a daily basis. Instead, you should focus on constructing an overall picture of your blood sugar every three or four months. When taking the fasting blood sugar, you should take your blood sugar on three different mornings and then average the results. This will help you to get a true picture of where your blood sugar stands.

It is also advisable to determine your body's response after a meal. You can do this with different foods, but for the purposes of determining whether or not you have problems with high blood sugar, you are going to want to test your blood sugar after consuming a meal that has a significant amount of carbohydrates. So you might want to test your blood sugar after eating a slice of pizza or a plate of pasta. Or simply test it after consuming what you normally eat, but of course, if you are going something like following a keto diet, you are not likely to see much of a reaction after consuming a meal that has low levels of carbohydrates.

Target Ranges

The first thing to think about is the type of blood sugar test you are doing. This is going to impact the target range that will determine where you stand. Let's consider the following scenarios.

Fasting

When testing fasting glucose, you want to see a blood glucose value in the range of 80-110 mg/dL for normal values. If it is slightly below this, then there really isn't much to worry about. As we noted earlier, a value of 54 mg/dL or less is a health emergency, but if your fasting level is 70 mg/dL and you feel fine, there is nothing to worry about.

If you get a slightly elevated value, our recommendation is to do a repeat test. You should do at least three tests and then average the results together, making sure that you fasted 8-12 hours before doing the test.

Testing After Eating

Testing after eating is going to be an important metric of the state of your health. First off, you need to keep careful track of what you are doing in this case. You don't want to test too early, because that will give you a false impression. It can take time for your blood sugar to reach its peak value. What you want to look for here is the peak value and how long it takes to see your blood sugar go back down. This is obviously only something you are going to be doing once in a while and not on a daily basis.

You should wait until at least one hour has passed since eating, and then take the first test. You should be recording the values you get in a notebook or on a spreadsheet on your computer or something to that effect. The details are not important, but you need to keep records to ensure accuracy. So record the time that you finished eating, and then the time of each successive blood test, and the reading at each time.

Next, take a second reading two hours after eating. For many people taking these two readings may be enough to get a good idea of how your body is responding to the consumption of carbohydrates. However, you might want to keep repeating the test at 30-minute intervals until your blood sugar returns back to the baseline value that you normally see with fasting glucose testing.

In most cases, a healthy person will not see their blood sugar go above 125 or 130 mg/dL after a meal, but even a result as high as 140 mg/dL is not too concerning. You should be concerned if you see very high spikes, and this would be on the order of 180 mg/dL or higher. Some people who are actually diabetic might see values go as high as 300 mg/dL or more.

A1C Testing At Home

In recent years, at home, A1C test kits have become available. We can't get into the details of using them at home because instructions will vary by manufacturer. Typically, an A1C kit will have to test kits per package. Fasting is not required for an A1C test, so you can do the test at any time, and the results will be reliable. Again, cutting corners with something like this is not something that you want to do, so you probably want to make sure you spend an extra $10 or $20 and get a test kit made by a reliable manufacturer.

You can use the kit in one of two ways. One way is to use both test devices at once so that you can average or confirm and be sure that you got an accurate reading. Alternatively, you can save one test device to use later, in three months after you have taken the test. If you obtain a result of 5.7% or less, this is an indication that your blood sugar is well controlled.

If you get a result between 5.8% and 6.4%, you can focus on diet, exercise, and losing weight to help get your blood sugar under control. If it is higher than this, you are probably best off contacting your doctor to discuss the results. They will probably want to confirm with their own test which is supposedly more accurate.

When to Contact Your Doctor

If you see results that are normal, then you don't need to worry. Just track your results and test again in a few months. If you do see high blood sugar readings, if your fasting glucose is less than 125 mg/dL, you can make changes in diet and exercise at home. You can also focus on losing weight if you are overweight or obese.

If you have high spikes that are concerning or high fasting blood sugar levels, it will be appropriate to visit your doctor and discuss the results. They will probably want to confirm with tests of their own to find out where your health stands and then take appropriate action. If you have spikes of 180 or higher or fasting blood glucose levels above 135, this is definitely not something to play around with, because untreated diabetes can have serious impacts on your health. That said, if you are in that situation, you can take treatments from your doctor to help you get your blood sugar under control, and then work on natural treatments to help get yourself off the medication over time.

For the A1C test, contact your doctor if you have a result of 6.5% or above if you have never done the test before. If you had gotten the test at your doctor before and had high results in the diabetic range, then it is not necessary to contact your doctor unless you are seeing your results increasing with time.

By keeping track of your fasting blood sugar and your A1C levels at home, you can get a solid picture of your blood sugar. If you are not diabetic, then there is nothing to worry about. People who might benefit from such testing are those with a family history of diabetes, or if you have had high blood sugar problems in the past that you are trying to manage using natural methods. While I prefer natural methods based on diet, lifestyle, and exercise, it is important to avoid being reckless. That is, you don't want to be avoiding going to the doctor when you should go to the doctor. Remember that in the event you do get put on medication, there are always going to be methods that you can use in order to reverse the condition, but it is important to not let high blood sugar go untreated. Any time that you are going around with high blood sugars that are not properly managed, and you can't manage them at home, you are putting yourself and your health at serious risk.

Low Blood Sugar Treatment

If you are finding that you have low blood sugar, the best way to treat it is to eat! Low blood sugar might also be dealt with by changing your diet. Your body might digest carbohydrates more rapidly than average, or maintain at lower blood sugar values. You can try working on a diet that has lower levels of carbohydrates and more fat for energy. But whether or not slightly low blood sugar values are a problem really depends on how you feel. If you feel fine, chances are this is not something to worry about at all. Remember the cutoffs for an emergency situation, and if your blood sugar is always above 70 mg/dL and you feel good and healthy and have enough energy, this is really not a problem. If your blood sugar gets low enough to be close to emergency levels, eat something with carbohydrates in it to raise your blood sugar back. It can help to eat something with simple sugars like a chocolate candy bar or drink some orange juice. Keep in mind that if you have a hypoglycemic episode, you might still feel hungry even after eating a large amount of calories, so don't overdo it. Eat a reasonable amount of sugar and see how you feel in 15 or 20 minutes.

High Blood Sugar Treatment

If your blood sugar is mildly elevated, engage in some aerobic exercise for at least 30 minutes, and avoid eating high carbohydrate foods. If you get hungry, eat an avocado or some fatty meat. Fatty fish is good to eat to give you energy without impacting your blood sugar. If your blood sugars go above 200 but are under 300, you should see a doctor, but a visit to the emergency room isn't necessary. Just monitor your blood sugar to see how it is developing with the passage of time, and you should probably see it start to drop. If this happens, however, a visit with your doctor for an evaluation is necessary.

If your blood sugar gets very high, you might need to visit an emergency room. Blood sugars of 400 mg/dL or above, can lead to a serious medical condition called ketoacidosis. This is not to be confused with ketosis, which is a normal and healthy process. In ketoacidosis, the body goes into an emergency mode because the cells are not able to utilize the glucose in the bloodstream. Ketones are released into the blood at unhealthy levels, leading to acidic conditions in the blood. Confusion, nausea, and vomiting can result, along with other symptoms like stomach pain.

Someone who is not yet diabetic, even if they routinely experience high blood sugar levels, is not going to experience ketoacidosis. You only need to worry about this if you have already been diagnosed as diabetic or if you have high blood sugar levels in the diabetic range, but your diabetes has never been treated. You should be concerned if you sometimes get blood sugar levels that are higher than 300 mg/dL after eating.

apter 4: Diseases Associated with High Blood Sugar

In this chapter, we are going to describe the main diseases associated with high blood sugar. There are two types of diabetes: the main type that appears in adulthood and can be controlled via diet and exercise is called type 2 diabetes. We will learn the difference between the two different types of diabetes and how to deal with it.

Type 1 and Type 2 Diabetes

One of the distinctions that people should be aware of is type 1 versus type 2 diabetes. Most readers of this book who are suffering from high blood sugar are at risk of type 2 diabetes. Type 1 diabetes typically happens in childhood or young adulthood, and it is due to a genetic susceptibility. In type 1 diabetes, it can be described as an autoimmune disorder. What happens is the body's immune system mistakenly destroys the cells in the pancreas that create insulin. Since the body can no longer make its own insulin, diabetes manifests as a disease.

This is an entirely different phenomenon as compared to type 2 diabetes. Certainly, there can be tendencies toward type 2 diabetes, and the susceptibility to it can run in families. But unlike type 1 diabetes, type 2 diabetes is directly related to the amount of body weight and body fat a person carries, how much they exercise, and what their diet is.

Type 1 diabetes is far more rare, and it is not amenable to the types of prescriptions that are laid out in this book. You can think of type 2 diabetes as something that we can cure with lifestyle and diet changes, but type 1 diabetes is not suitable for these types of changes. In short, type 1 diabetes is a disease that is only going to be handled by supplemental insulin because the immune system has destroyed the very cells that produce insulin in the body.

In contrast, type 2 diabetes is a lifestyle disease, regardless of how much is inherited. It is true that some people are more susceptible to the sugar content of foods than others, but no matter how sensitive you are, type 2 diabetes is something that can definitely be monitored and controlled through the type of diet and lifestyle that you follow in your life.

One key difference between the two diseases is that in type 1 diabetes, the beta cells in the pancreas that make insulin are destroyed. So the bottom line with type 1 diabetes is the body cannot make insulin. It must be supplied through external sources, and there is no cure that can be manifest through changes in lifestyle, diet, exercise, or weight loss.

In contrast, with type 2 diabetes, the body can make plenty of insulin. However, the body is no longer sensitive to the effects of insulin. So while type 1 diabetes is a genetic or autoimmune disease involving the lack of insulin, type 2 diabetes is a disease where there is plenty of insulin produced by the body (at least at first), but the body does not respond to normal levels of insulin. Another way to put this is type 1 diabetes is a disease of insulin deprivation, while type 2 diabetes is a disease whereby the body is not sensitive to insulin.

Age of Diagnosis

Type 1 diabetes is typically diagnosed in children or young adults. In contrast, type 2 diabetes is usually diagnosed in middle-aged adults. In recent years, more and more people are getting diagnosed with type 2 diabetes at younger ages, but this is a result of lifestyle changes. People are less active than they used to be, and they are having more problems with obesity at younger ages. These problems are at the result of insulin resistance, and although type 1 and type 2 diabetes are different at a fundamental level, the clinical manifestations of both diseases are the same.

The causes of type 1 diabetes are well-known. In short, it is an autoimmune disease. There are certain cells in the pancreas called beta cells that produce insulin in the body. In type 1 diabetes, these cells are attacked by the immune system, and so the patient is left without the ability to produce insulin. It is an insulin production disease.

In contrast, with type 2 diabetes, there is no autoimmune component, and insulin is still produced. Type 2 diabetes is instead a lifestyle disease. It is related to physical inactivity, weight gain, and poor dietary choices. Age and family history may also be related to type 2 diabetes.

Symptoms

Even though the causes are very different, the symptoms are the same. To understand why, let's try to imagine what happens at a fundamental level. With type 1 diabetes, the cells that make insulin in the body are destroyed, and so no or little insulin is produced. The result of this is that blood sugar rises to out of control levels, and the cells are unable to take up blood sugar to use in the body.

When blood sugar levels rise in type 1 diabetes, the high blood sugar levels have the same impact on the body, as they do when type 1 diabetes is not present. They will destroy small blood vessels and capillaries, resulting in damage to the body's organs and tissues.

In type 2 diabetes, although insulin is produced, at least in the early stages, it has no impact on the cells that are no longer sensitive to it. As a result, there is a buildup of blood sugar. So although the root causes of type 2 diabetes are very different, the end result is the same. In both cases, you have cells that are unable to take up the sugar that is present in the blood. This means that the cells are going to be low on energy in both cases because they are unable to even access it. Secondly, high blood sugars will result in the same damage to organs and the circulatory system in both cases.

So if type 1 or type 2 diabetes are left untreated, the same symptoms and complications can develop. A type 1 diabetic is going to suffer from low energy and fatigue, high blood sugar and dehydration and thirst accompanied by high amounts of urination. They are also going to suffer from many of the other common problems like vision problems, slow healing of wounds, and kidney problems. Thirst and hunger are also present in both cases.

Diagnosis

Diabetes will be diagnosed using multiple blood tests. The first indication of diabetes is a high fasting blood sugar. Generally, a reading of 125 mg/dL or higher after 8-12 hours of fasting is taken to indicate diabetes is present. However, a single reading is not definitive for diagnosis. Two or more readings with a result in this range can indicated diabetes is present and indicate further testing.

This information will be evaluated in conjunction with any symptoms that you describe to the doctor, such as fatigue, chronic thirst, and frequent urination. No single item on this list is definitive, but by considering everything along with a few tests, a comprehensive picture can be built to determine the state of health regarding blood sugar and diabetes.

If your doctor finds that you have two or more readings with a fasting blood sugar level of 125 mg/dL or higher, they will order a glucose tolerance test. This will help determine your body's response to glucose in real-time, allowing the doctor to determine how high your blood sugar will peak after consuming carbohydrates. In addition, the doctor will want to have some idea of how long it takes your blood sugar to return to the baseline or background level seen with the fasting test. The way your body responds to the glucose tolerance test can be taken together with the fasting blood glucose level in order to determine if you have a diagnosis of diabetes.

When it comes to an official diagnosis of diabetes, the A1C test is considered the gold standard. To understand why you can go back to the discussion we had earlier about the test – the A1C test allows the doctor to determine your average blood sugar over the past 90 days. This gives a complete picture of how your body handles blood sugar than either a fasting glucose test or a glucose tolerance test. If the A1C is 6.5% or higher, this results in a diagnosis of diabetes. Many people with diabetes will have A1C values that are much higher than this, even in the 7-11% range. Therefore, don't panic if you have an A1C value that is in the range of 6.5-7%. You might still be able to get your condition under control without having to resort to medication.

Dealing with Type 2 versus Type 1 Diabetes

The main difference between type 1 and type 2 diabetes is that type 1 diabetes is not amenable to lifestyle changes. If a patient has type 1 diabetes, he or she must take insulin, because the lack of insulin is the main factor in the disease. In contrast, while insulin must be administered in some and (usually) in more advanced cases, most of the time, type 2 diabetes is very susceptible to changes in diet and exercise.

In either case, if the disease is untreated, heart disease, stroke, cancer, and amputation are among the many complications that can result from the disease. In both cases, there is a susceptibility to diabetic ketoacidosis.

Obesity and Diabetes

When it comes to type 1 diabetes, low body mass rather than high body mass is likely to be a problem. In most cases, if you are already in adulthood, the closer you are to middle age, the more likely it is that you are not suffering from type 1 diabetes if you are showing symptoms. Most people in adulthood who have not had diabetes up until this point are going to be suffering from type 2 diabetes.

When it comes to type 2 diabetes, there are three factors that stand out. These are obesity, activity levels, and dietary choices. At the root of these problems is insulin resistance, which is a situation where the cells do not respond to a given level of insulin in a normal manner. Insulin leads to weight gain because one of the roles that insulin plays in the body is it causes excess blood sugar to be converted into fat, which is then pushed into storage by the body via insulin. When someone is insulin resistant, this means that they are going to be carrying around more blood sugar in their system, to begin with, and so it is more likely to be stored as body fat. So, in short, diabetes or a tendency toward diabetes is going to result in insulin resistance, which means there are going to be higher levels of blood sugar. In turn, this means that this blood sugar is more likely to be turned into body fat. The increased levels of body fat will then lead to even more problems with insulin resistance, creating a negative and unhealthy cycle.

When distinguishing between type 1 and type 2 diabetes, note that obesity is rarely associated with type 1 diabetes, but it is commonly associated with type 2 diabetes. However, in either case, it is important to maintain a proper body weight once you have been diagnosed as diabetic, no matter what the ultimate cause is.

Lack of Exercise, Poor Diet and Diabetes

Once again, type1 diabetes is largely a genetic condition and an autoimmune disease. However, type 2 diabetes is largely a lifestyle disease. Two of the factors that are very important in the development of type 2 diabetes are lack of exercise and poor diet. A lack of exercise is definitely related to the development of diabetes, either right now or in the future.

Diet is one of those things that you can have a significant if not total means of control of. When you have diabetes, you can choose to change your diet. In future chapters, we will talk about the impact that diet has on diabetes. The fewer carbohydrates that you consume in your diet, the less likely it is that you are going to end up becoming or maintaining diabetes.

Exercise is closely related to the development of diabetes, and if you are already diagnosed with diabetes, the lack of exercise is generally associated with poor outcomes. Exercise helps to condition all the body's cells to take up insulin in order to satisfy their energy needs. This is definitely true for the large muscle groups, but it is also true for any cells in the body, no matter their type or location. Think about the way that your body becomes active during exercise, and how it will take up blood sugar in order to satisfy the energy needs of the individual cells and clear out and use up what energy sources it has available already.

Chapter 5: Causes and Symptoms

The natural state of the body is one that includes just the right level of sugar in the blood. Your body is already accustomed to this, and it instinctively knows how much it needs. Systems in the bodywork to ensure that blood sugar does not dip below a minimum value, which would lead to mental confusion, loss of consciousness, and possibly a state of coma. However, those systems can break down. Alternatively, when the body is in a totally dysfunctional state because of diabetes that is untreated, blood sugar can rise so high that it creates a health crisis.

Blood sugar gives the body's cells and organs all of the energy that is needed for proper functioning. If the right amount of blood sugar is not present or more to the point for our purposes, the cells cannot take up that blood sugar; then problems are going to be the immediate result. In most cases, the results are not going to be as dramatic as those described above, and sugar is only going to be mildly elevated.

Poor Memory and Low Energy

Poor memory and low energy are two symptoms to look out for as an adult, when it comes to the manifestations of high blood sugar or blood sugar that is not properly managed by the body, leading to excessive highs or lows. When your blood sugars are such that they are routinely low, or your body is having problems using the blood sugar that is there, right in the body, you are going to be lacking in energy and showing many of the basic symptoms of diabetes discussed in detail in the last chapter. These include:

- High levels of thirst
- Excessive urination
- A constant sensation of dehydration
- Possible vision problems
- Numbness and tingling
- High blood sugar
- High blood pressure
- Heart disease
- Stroke

Who would want to endure all of these problems? I am sure that most of us would agree that taking on all of the health conditions that are related to high blood sugar is not something most of us would want to deal with.

Let's consider fatigue and low energy. When you have high blood sugar, the glucose molecules that provide energy for your cells are not taken up in adequate amounts. This means that your cells are constantly running low on fuel. The net result is that your body is going to be in a low energy state at all times, and even eating large meals is never going to get you out of this state. Many people are suffering low energy without realizing that high blood sugar is the culprit. As we described earlier, the high levels of blood sugar are the result of insulin resistance, whereby the cells are no longer responding to the signals given by insulin to open up and take in the blood sugar. Think of it as working at a job where you used to work hard for $10 an hour, but as you get older and less experienced, you're not going to be willing to put in the same amount of work unless you are paid $20 an hour. So it takes more money to get you to put in the same amount of time and effort to work. Likewise, when it comes to the body and blood sugar, it takes more insulin to get the cells to take up the same amount of glucose. Over time, just like your boss might run out of money if you keep needing a raise to do the same job, the body is unable to keep up with demands for insulin, and so the cells are basically in an underfed state.

When you are not able to take in all the available energy from the glucose circulating in your system, your brain is going to get a double whammy. In short, the brain will not function as well due to your overall problem of low energy. We all know that if we are not properly nourished and well-rested, we simply can't function as well mentally. But the brain is also going to have problems properly utilizing blood sugar since under these conditions; you are going to have insulin resistance – so even the brain cells are not going to be able to take in the proper amount of sugar. That means that your mental capacity is going to be taken down a couple of notches, putting you in a sort of brain fog. You might attribute the brain fog to feeling tired, not realizing that high blood sugar is the cause. Poor memory may be one of the results that you experience when you are not able to fully function and extract all of the energy from the meals you consume. This is one reason that it is important to get your blood sugar tested on a regular basis so that you don't end up suffering severe consequences from high blood sugar that is not corrected.

Causes of Type 2 Diabetes

Before we discuss some of the causes that are believed to contribute to type 2 diabetes, it is important to remind the reader that type 1 diabetes is a different disease, although the symptoms and final stage results are the same. To remind readers, type 1 diabetes results when insulin-producing cells in the pancreas are destroyed. This can be an autoimmune disease or may possibly be the result of a viral disease or some other infection. Type 1 diabetes is something acquired during childhood or adolescence. This is different from type 2 diabetes. Although type 2 diabetes definitely comes with a genetic component that can give someone a tendency to get it, it is largely a disease of lifestyle. This is not to blame anyone who has it. In part, the culture we are embedded in gives many of us a tendency to get type 2 diabetes because of the prevailing dietary and exercise habits. Nonetheless, type 2 diabetes can be traced to the amount of food you eat, the amount and types of carbohydrates that you consume, and the amount of exercise you get along with a few other factors. Many if not most of these factors are under our control.

The Role of Food in Type 2 Diabetes

The most fundamental factor in the development of type 2 diabetes is the kind of food you eat. How responsive you are to different foods and whether or not they lead you to develop type 2 diabetes is going to be something that is related to your family history, and also to your other habits such as the amount and quality of sleep and exercise. Nonetheless, food is probably the biggest factor, and it is possible to control, prevent, and even reverse diabetes by changing your diet. The degree to which you need to change your diet is going to vary from one individual to the next, and this is determined by family history. You will have to decide for yourself how far you are willing to go in order to avoid medication and control the condition naturally, but in many, if not most cases, it can be controlled naturally.

Total Carbohydrates

Some people are simply not suited for eating large amounts of carbohydrates in their diet. This is true no matter how many whole grains are consumed or whether or not there are high or low glycemic foods consumed. In this case, a low carb or ketogenic diet should be considered. One fact that has been verified scientifically and medically is that a ketogenic diet can prevent, reverse, or at least control type 2 diabetes in all cases. But you may not want to eat a ketogenic diet. There are many variations of this approach that can be tried, and the best thing to do is try a given diet for 3 months, and then take an A1C test to see what the impact of the diet was on your blood sugar. If you start with a mildly low carb diet and it does not work for you, then you should try a more restricted approach.

Paleo Diet

The mildest form of low carb diet is known as the paleo diet. This type of diet is going to eliminate any bread or carbohydrate-based products that were invented using civilization. In other words, you will not consume any bread, crackers, cookies, cake, pasta, or other kinds of carbohydrate-based foods. However, on the paleo diet you are allowed to consume most natural sources of carbohydrates. So you can eat fruit and consume sweet potatoes (but adherents do not consume plain potatoes). This is not a diet book, and so a detailed description of a given diet is beyond the scope of this book, but think of the diet as fruit, vegetables, and meat. Any type of meat item is allowed, including all the basics like beef, poultry, pork, and fish, but the preference is for meat in the most natural state possible, so free range is preferred. You can also use regular butter, but most paleo adherents generally avoid dairy.

Atkins/Low Carb

If the paleo diet is not able to reverse your high blood sugar, the next step would probably be something like the Atkins diet. This diet is divided up into phases and emphasizes the consumption of fatty meat and vegetables. In the first phase, which lasts a couple of weeks, carbohydrates are limited to 20 net carbohydrates per day. A net carbohydrate is found by taking the total carbohydrates in a given food and subtracting the fiber. As time goes on, at successive stages you can keep increasing the amount of carbohydrates consumed. You are never going to return to a "standard" level of carbohydrate consumption, but you might be able to consume 100-150 grams of carbohydrates per day. The goal is to reverse course if you find you start gaining weight again.

Ketogenic Diet

In recent years, the ketogenic diet has become very popular. It is also very effective at controlling diabetes, and many adherents to the keto diet are able to reverse prediabetes and diabetes or prevent it if they have a family history. It is also very effective at generating weight loss, although the paleo and Atkins diets are able to generate large amounts of weight loss for many people as well. The keto diet is fat-based and relies on putting the body in a state of ketosis so that it gets most of its energy from fat rather than from sugar. Your body will still maintain normal blood sugar levels in ketosis, but even the brain will get 70% of its energy from fat when you are in this state. Do not confuse this with ketoacidosis; the ketosis state is perfectly natural and healthy. By following a keto diet for several months, many dieters are able to completely reset their blood sugar system and eliminate insulin resistance.

The diet is largely fat rather than protein-based. However, a typical meal will include meat and green vegetables. You can eat avocados liberally because most of the carbohydrates in avocadoes are from dietary fiber. The goal is to consume 75-80% of your calories from fat, 15-20% from protein, and 5% from carbohydrates. You are allowed to eat as many green vegetables as you want on a diet, so it is not a meat-based diet.

Intermittent Fasting

Every night when you sleep, your body actually enters a state where it could go into ketosis. This is caused by another hormone made by the pancreas called glucagon. This hormone releases body fat that has been stored so it can be broken down into ketones and used as fuel. Glucagon also causes glycogen (stored carbohydrate) in the liver to be used up. When glucagon levels are high, insulin levels are low. This means that intermittent fasting is something good for people with insulin resistance and high insulin levels to use to help reset their body to a healthier state. Fasting can be done in a variety of ways, and it can be used in conjunction with any type of diet. One of the most popular ways to use intermittent fasting is the so-called 16/8 method. You simply confine your eating to an eight hour time period each day. Many prediabetics and diabetics have reported amazing results using this method. The more diabetic you are, that is, the higher your A1C and fasting glucose levels, the more restrictive you should be. One way to do this is only eating one meal per day. That is not a calorie-restricted method; you are expected to consume all of your daily calories requirements within one hour. That is too much for people, though, so you could consider splitting it into two meals only spaced 4-6 hours apart or simply using 16/8 fasting with a restricted keto diet. If you have been diagnosed with diabetes and are on medication, consult with your doctor before making major changes to your diet or using fasting methods.

Glycemic Index

It is not necessary to give up carbohydrate-based foods, but you will have to do what works for your situation. If you are able to control your blood sugar without giving up carbohydrates, the best way to do it is to pay attention to the types of carbohydrates that you are consuming. The goal here is to aim for carbohydrates that cause a slower rise in blood sugar after consuming the food. These are foods with a low glycemic index. Typically, this type of food is going to have a higher component of dietary fiber, combined with longer chains of carbohydrates. This will mean that the food takes a longer amount of time to digest. Virtually all doctors are in agreement that patients who have high blood sugar should consume foods with a low glycemic index.

When you consume sugar, it will result in a very rapid rise in your blood sugar to a high peak value. Then it will take a long time for your blood sugar to drop back down to the baseline range. When you are making comparisons between different foods to learn the glycemic index, you can consider the consumption of pure sugar as the worst-case scenario.

In contrast, a complex carbohydrate with a large amount of dietary fiber will take longer to digest. It takes time for the body to break apart all the molecules so that the individual glucose molecules can be liberated and released into the bloodstream. As a result, in theory at least, blood sugar will rise gradually, and since the rise is gradual, it is spread out over a long time period, and it will peak at a lower level than what you would see with sugar or sugary type foods. This is a more healthy pattern for blood sugar since lower peak values mean that there is less damage to the blood vessels and organ systems of the body.

A diet which is based on foods with a good glycemic diet is claimed to produce weight loss when used in conjunction with a reduced-calorie regimen. It is also effective at simply helping you maintain your current weight while allowing you to plan healthy meals that are balanced among all of the major food groups. If you are prediabetic or diabetic, a diet that is based on the glycemic index is going to help you maintain your blood sugar levels within a healthier range. In most cases, however, it will probably not allow diabetics to get off their medication, although you might be able to reduce dosages. If you use a diet based on the glycemic index you might be able to reduce or get off medications if you lose a significant amount of weight.

The glycemic index is a score assigned to each food item that ranges from 1 to 100+. The higher the score, the more the impact of the food on your blood sugar. The glycemic index is split into three general categories:

- Low Glycemic Index: The range for low glycemic foods is 1 to 55. These are the best foods to eat for maintaining healthy blood sugar levels and avoiding dangerous spikes.
- Medium Glycemic Index: A medium-range is 56-69. Foods in this category can be consumed in moderation, but should not be consumed too frequently. On most days you should avoid foods with a medium glycemic index.
- High Glycemic Index: These are foods that have a glycemic index of 70 and above. These foods are high impact when it comes to blood sugar and should be avoided most of the time, and depending on the severity of your condition, you may choose to completely avoid them. When you are thinking in terms of high glycemic foods, think white bread, honey, sugar, and molasses.

The goal of assigning a glycemic index to each food item is to make it easy for prediabetics and diabetics to select food items that will have minimal impact on their blood sugar. It is important to avoid using a low glycemic index as a license to eat large portions of food.

Drawbacks of the Glycemic Index

Maintaining a healthy weight is critical when it comes to keeping your blood sugar in healthy ranges, and even though a food might be healthy when it comes to the glycemic index, you can still gain weight if you eat outsized portions. Another drawback of focusing entirely on the glycemic index is that you don't get any information about the nutritional content of the food. It only conveys the response of the body to the food in terms of blood sugar values. A processed food that has little nutritional value, and might be high in salt and fat, could have a low glycemic index. That could mean it is not the most healthy food for you to consume if you are looking to lose or maintain your current weight.

Another drawback when it comes to the glycemic index is that the quantity of food typically consumed is not really reflected in the real-world impact on a person's blood sugar level. For example, watermelon is often used to illustrate this because it has a high glycemic index at 80. However, watermelon is not calorie-dense. In other words, you would not be digesting very much carbohydrate, eating a slice of watermelon. So in practice, it is not going to raise your blood sugar very much. But if you are a glutton, and you eat an entire watermelon, you will get a significant carb load and find that you have a big rise in blood sugar.

Methods of food preparation can also impact the way that a food will affect your blood sugar levels. Cooking food can break down some of the components, making it easier to digest. In practice, this can mean that the food might have more of an impact on your blood sugar when cooked. You should look into what state of the food is reflected by a specific glycemic index if applicable.

A note on low carb diets and glycemic index

Meats, fish, and fats have a glycemic index of zero. Many foods included on low carb diets like avocados, nuts, and leafy green vegetables are very low in carbohydrate, and so have a minimal if any impact on blood sugar. In fact, the impact on blood sugar is so low that researchers haven't even bothered to determine the glycemic index of avocados. You can also take it to be zero. If you are following a ketogenic diet, you are probably going to find that your blood sugar barely changes, if it changes at all, after eating a large meal.

Examples of Glycemic Index

For those who are interested in trying a diet based on the glycemic index, let's have a look at the glycemic index of some popular foods. This can be an eye-opening exercise because some foods that you would consider healthy actually have a high glycemic index. For example, when it comes to your blood sugar, what do you think is better, white spaghetti, a corn tortilla, or whole wheat bread? White spaghetti has a glycemic index of about 49. A corn tortilla checks in a little bit better at 46, but whole wheat bread is a high glycemic index food – meaning that it has more impact on blood sugar. It checks in with a glycemic index of 74.

Rice noodles and udon noodles are even better than whole wheat bread, with a glycemic index of 55. Specialty grain bread is much better than standard whole wheat bread. In that case, the glycemic index is about 53.

Typically the glycemic index has a range of values and not one specific value. This is because not all examples of food are going to be exactly the same. For example, white spaghetti actually ranges from 47 to 51. It is often listed as having a glycemic index of 49 +/- 2.

Breakfast cereals tend to be high glycemic foods. The glycemic index of corn flakes is 81 +/- 6. That is a pretty high level, and it is interesting to contemplate the long term impact on health that corn flakes have had since their introduction into the American diet in the early 20ᵗʰ century.

Whole fruits are fairly decent when it comes to the glycemic index. An apple has one of the lowest glycemic indices among fruits, with a value of 36. A whole orange is 43, while orange juice is 50. Most fruits fall somewhere in the range of 40-50. It is important to keep in mind that while fruits are a great source of many of the vitamins, minerals, and antioxidants that we need, studies have shown that they are not necessarily healthy when consumed in large amounts. Remember that the regular consumption of orange juice has been proven to increase triglyceride levels significantly, which means that orange juice can actually increase the risk of heart disease in some people. If you are going to eat fruit, you should consume it in moderation if you have problems with high blood sugar. An alternative is to limit yourself to berries, which tend to contain fewer carbohydrates per serving, and they also have lower glycemic indexes. Examples include blueberries, strawberries, raspberries, and blackberries.

Now let's look at vegetables. Start with the potato, which is basically just a starch factory. The glycemic index of white mashed potatoes is 87, a very high value. It is practically the same as consuming pure sugar. A boiled potato is a little better at 78. French fries are even better at 63, the same glycemic index as a boiled sweet potato.

When it comes to milk, the type of milk consumed doesn't seem to matter much. Whole milk actually has a slightly higher glycemic index than skim milk, but the differences are negligible at 39 and 37. That means these are low glycemic foods. Ice cream has a glycemic index of 51. Soy milk is similar to cows' milk, but there are reasons to avoid consuming soy milk because it contains plant estrogens, which impact the body in the same way that estrogens do. Rice milk has a very high glycemic index at 86.

Beans and legumes all have low glycemic indexes and have high amounts of fiber. The same holds true for nuts.

Glycemic Index Obviously Doesn't Tell the Whole Story

Some foods that are clearly not good for you have a low glycemic index. For example, a soft drink has a glycemic index of 59, which is quite a bit lower than say a boiled potato. Do you think your health is better off eating a boiled potato -which contains potassium and vitamin C or drinking a soda?

Another example is fructose, which has a low glycemic index at 15, according to the Harvard Health Newsletter. Despite the low glycemic index, fructose is known to be very damaging to the body if you are prediabetic or diabetic. For reference, glucose has a glycemic index of 103, and ordinary table sugar (sucrose) has a glycemic index of 63. That is the same as a sweet potato, which is loaded with dietary fiber and vitamin A. Do you think a sweet potato or three tablespoons of table sugar are better for your health? These examples show that while the glycemic index is useful to a point, it should not be the last word in determining your dietary choices. The whole food must be considered.

How to Eat to Control Your Blood Sugar

The best way to control your blood sugar, in the event you are not following a low carbohydrate diet, is to eat balanced meals. Besides noting the glycemic index, one factor that can influence the way that your blood sugar is going to respond to consuming a particular food is what else you eat with it. If you eat a tablespoon of sugar, it is probably going to have more impact on your blood sugar than it would if it was in a sauce that was on a piece of salmon, for example. Consuming a reasonable amount of protein with your meal is going to help you to have better control over your blood sugar, as opposed to consuming carbohydrates in isolation. Fat will also slow the absorption of any sugars that you consume in a meal, helping you avoid the high blood sugar spikes that are so worrisome when it comes to overall health.

Another factor that is very important when considering eating to control your blood sugar is the amount of dietary fiber consumed in each meal.

The amount of dietary fiber in a food is known to have an impact on the glycemic index of a food, and the total amount of dietary fiber in each meal is also going to have an impact on the overall impact on your blood sugar caused by the meal, not just the individual food items that you consume. When possible, always opt to include foods that have high dietary fiber content as a part of your overall diet plan.

Incorporating vegetables with every meal can also help. Most vegetables, with the exception of potatoes and sweet potatoes, are foods that have a low glycemic index, and they also have a high amount of dietary fiber. The large fiber content can make your meals more filling, and so including large servings of vegetables will help you control portion sizes of calorie-dense foods in your meals such as meat and bread. In addition, vegetables contain many chemicals that medical researchers believe have anti-cancer properties. So not only will including a large amount of vegetables help you manage your blood sugar more effectively, they will also help you to fight off disease. And at the same time, vegetables can help you put together more tasty dishes.

Focus on including so-called good fats in your meals. Adding fat to meals, paradoxically, can help you to lose weight. The reason that this happens is fat in your meals will make them more satisfying, and so you will eat smaller portion sizes overall. Consider adding a half an avocado to each of your meals. Avocados not only contain a large amount of dietary fiber, along with important vitamins and minerals like vitamin C and potassium, they also contain large amounts of monounsaturated fats. The evidence that these types of fats are actually good for you is overwhelming. Consuming large amounts of monounsaturated fats has been proven to reduce the risk of heart disease and stroke, and since diabetics are at elevated risk of developing heart disease, it makes sense to consume foods that are rich in monounsaturated fats. Again, the increased calorie and energy density of foods like avocados will actually mean you are able to have more satisfying meals while consuming smaller portions. So you can actually lose weight by consuming more fat.

Olive oil is another fat that should be included in the dietary habits of those who are looking to get better control of their blood sugar. Like avocado, olives contain high levels of monounsaturated fats. Olive oil is unmatched, except by the consumption of fatty fish, when it comes to reducing the risk of heart disease. Adding olive oil to your meals will also help enrich the flavors and make them more satisfying. This will help you to keep your blood sugar under better control.

Another option for those who like the taste is to eat a lot of fatty fish. Fatty fish contains helpful omega-3 oils, which are known to help lower triglycerides and reduce the risk of developing heart disease. Those who consume large amounts of fatty fish are also known to have a lower risk of sudden death from heart attack. We have already discussed the many benefits and noted that salmon, mackerel, tuna, anchovies, trout, and several other fatty fish are good to consume for heart health. For our purposes here, we want to note that consuming fatty fish in your meals is another way to make the meal seem more "solid" and satisfying. When you eat solid food that is rich in fat and protein, you are going to be able to get more energy out of smaller portions. The net result of this is that you are going to be consuming fewer calories overall, and this will help you maintain or lose weight, which means better control over your blood sugar over the long-term. Even in the short-term, since the addition of fatty fish to your meals will help to make them more satisfying, you are going to find that your blood sugar is better controlled.

The use of artificial sweeteners is controversial to some, so it is up to the individual to do their own research and decide whether or not to use them. Splenda is the best one to use, but it should be used in moderation. Surprisingly, artificial sweeteners have been found to actually raise the blood sugar of people using them in large amounts. However, if they are used in moderation to sweeten drinks like coffee or tea, they should not have much if any impact on your blood sugar.

The Best Way Forward : Experiment

It is one thing to look up the glycemic index of a given food, and try to plan out your diet. The best thing to do is gather some actual data. If you are already monitoring your blood sugar at home, this is very easy to do. Use the procedure described to check your blood sugar after a meal for specific foods. So eat a potato and then take your blood sugar 1 hour and 2 hours after eating to see how *your* body responds to the consumption of potatoes. Even though each food is assigned an objective glycemic index, that doesn't mean that everyone is going to respond to different foods in the same way. Different individuals may be able to tolerate some foods more than others. And if you have the capacity to actually find out what a given food item is going to do when it comes to your blood sugar levels, why not actually test it and find out? You can build up your own little database of foods you can eat and foods to avoid, by recording what levels your blood sugar reaches after consuming them in isolation. So to avoid complicating things, eat a potato by itself (or a slice of bread, a cup of ice cream, or whatever it may be) so that you can determine how your body responds to it. In addition to finding foods that you can eat without having too much impact on your blood sugar, you can use this method to also determine what foods to avoid when it comes to keeping your blood sugar under control.

Managing Your Sweet Tooth

Many of us have a sweet tooth, and one of the problems for those who are having problems with high blood sugar is that you might be in a situation where giving up sweet foods is going to be necessary. However, it is not always the case that you have to completely give up these foods, and there are ways to get around it.

The first thing to consider, however, is that you probably don't need to eat sweet foods nearly as much as you think you need to. One of the fears that people adopting a keto diet have, for example, is having to go without sweet foods most of the time, or even permanently. But like any addiction, when you make a break with the addicting substance, over time, your perceptions and tastes change. It may be hard to imagine now, but if you have a sweet tooth and go cold turkey, over time you are going to find that your cravings for sweet foods begin to go away. Pretty soon, you might even find that you don't need or want sweet-tasting foods at all. Some people might discover that after going several months without them, they even find them a bit repulsive.

Of course, extremes are not always necessary, and there are other ways to manage your sweet tooth without having to avoid sweet foods altogether. The first thing to recognize is that you are not going to blow your entire life or your health on one meal or food item. As long as you are not consuming sweet foods on a regular basis, they are not going to have a large impact on your overall health. Let's say that you like chocolate cake. Sure, eating chocolate cake daily is going to be bad for anyone's health, especially if you are prediabetic or diabetic. But eating chocolate cake once a week – that is something that is going to have far less impact. Eating it every two weeks, it will have even less impact. Eat it once a month, and it probably isn't going to influence your overall health at all.

I am not a big believer in forced deprivation, and I actually think that allowing yourself to indulge on occasion is going to be better for you in the long run. If you try and completely eliminate a favorite class of food, you are probably going to develop a massive craving for it, and end up splurging, binging, and overeating. In that case, you might find yourself routinely "ruining" your diet and damaging your health. For that reason, my feeling is that if you crave certain sweet foods, whether it's a candy bar or ice cream, allow yourself to enjoy it once a week or once every two weeks in moderation. Just don't get in a situation where you compile a list of 30 "forbidden" foods, and then find that you are eating one of them daily.

A good example of how to approach it is found in the book "4-hour body" by Timothy Ferris. He lost a large amount of weight by following a relatively low carb diet, but he allowed himself a cheat day once per week. On that day, he would eat everything he wanted, whether it was pizza, ice cream, or cake. The rest of the week, he would follow his rather strict diet, which limited the amount of carbohydrates consumed.

For those who have problems managing their blood sugar, the Ferris approach is probably not the best one to use. Once a week of eating everything you want is probably not going to be good for a prediabetic or diabetic, but the basic principle, setting aside a limited time to consume foods you crave – is something that most people can work into their routine without having a major impact on their health.

The best thing to do, always, is to test. Try something out and see how it impacts you by making real measurements. Check your average fasting blood sugar over the course of a month or two, and then incorporate a cheat day and see if that changes your average blood sugar. Also, watch your body weight. If you find that eating your favorite sweets once a week doesn't have any impact, great! You can continue following the diet and enjoy your sweets. However, if you find that your blood sugars are creeping up and you are gaining weight, then you know that you need to scale things back. Try only consuming sweets every two weeks instead. The point is to use actual data to arrive at a decision and to do what works for you. Every reader of this book is going to be different, and it's simply not possible to put together a one-size-fits-all plan. The reality is some people are going to be able to eat more sweets than others. Some are going to find that allowing themselves to consume sweets gets them into trouble, and they end up binging. Others are going to find that they can successfully enjoy sweets now and then.

Does eating sweets cause diabetes? It is not really possible to make that strong of a claim, but if you are genetically prone to developing type 2 diabetes, consuming a large amount of sweets, or even consuming sweets in moderation but on a regular basis, can tip the scales against you and cause you to develop type 2 diabetes. It is not possible to get around the fact that candy, ice cream, cake, and other sweet food items like donuts and pastries are going to cause blood sugar spikes. The more of these foods you consume, the more blood sugar spikes you are going to have, and the more likely it is you are going to develop insulin resistance. So in most people who are prone to develop prediabetes or type 2 diabetes because of family history, consuming sweets is something that is going to contribute to the development of disease, if not cause it outright.

Prescription Drug-Induced Diabetes

It is now clear that consuming certain drugs on a regular basis can cause diabetes. In some cases, the diabetes will go away. In other cases, unfortunately, diabetes may be permanent. Many drugs that can cause diabetes are legal, and some people may develop blood sugar problems while taking drugs on the advice of a doctor. One drug to watch out for is steroids. These can be abused, and one of the unfortunate side effects can be drug-induced diabetes. The consumption of steroids over a long time period can induce type 2 diabetes, and it is a permanent effect. This means that even if you stop taking the drugs, you are going to have type 2 diabetes the rest of your life. This can even happen when taking steroids at levels prescribed by your doctor, but if you are abusing steroids it may be even more likely because abusers of the drugs will be taking them at unhealthy levels and taking them when it is not necessary to take them.

Another legal class of drugs that can induce diabetes are statins. These are drugs that are commonly prescribed by doctors for the management of high cholesterol levels. The benefits of reducing risk by lowering cholesterol and other effects have to be weighed against the risk of inducing diabetes. Remember that diabetes in and of itself is a major risk factor for heart disease. Diabetics are known to be at twice the risk of having a heart attack, and they also have a higher risk of stroke. It doesn't make sense, if you are not having blood sugar problems, to put yourself at risk of developing them and triggering type 2 diabetes, and in the end, being at a much higher risk of having a heart attack. Statins now come with a warning of the risk of high blood sugars as a result of taking the drug. If you are already pre-diabetic or have a family history, you might want to use other methods of reducing your risk of heart disease rather than taking statins. At this time, it is not known if type 2 diabetes triggered by the intake of statins is permanent.

Type 2 diabetes can also be induced by diuretics. These are 'water pills' that are commonly prescribed for high blood pressure. Diuretics have many unpleasant side effects, such as depleting the body's supply of potassium, along with the sodium and excess fluids they are designed to get out of the body. They can also induce type 2 diabetes if used for long periods. In some cases, getting off the drugs will end the diabetes, but some people may find that they permanently have type 2 diabetes as a result of using diuretics.

Another legal medication that is quite commonly prescribed that can lead to the development of diabetes are beta-blockers. The most common reason they are prescribed is to control blood pressure. Beta-blockers can induce type 2 diabetes because they reduce insulin sensitivity.

Drug and Alcohol Addiction

Alcohol is not generally known to cause diabetes, but alcohol consumption for those with diabetes can have negative effects. And in some cases, if alcohol abuse is extensive, it can trigger type 2 diabetes. This may happen because of its impact on the liver and the pancreas, two organs that are closely related to maintaining a healthy blood sugar system.

The liver plays a central role in the management of blood sugar, and releasing blood sugar to maintain healthy levels in your bloodstream is one of the important jobs done by the liver. Alcohol can interfere with this process because the liver has to devote a lot of energy to process it. If consumed in significant amounts, alcohol can actually lead to low blood sugars, and a condition of hypoglycemia can result. Alcohol also has many impacts throughout the body, and diabetics are particularly sensitive to them. For example, diabetics will already have nerve damage throughout the body, and alcohol can worsen the impact of this nerve damage. In addition, if you are diabetic and you have developed eye problems; as a result, alcohol can make those worse as well.

Acute alcohol abuse can also trigger a condition called pancreatitis. Since the pancreas is where insulin is made by the body, this is not something that you want to have happen to you if you are already diabetic. Pancreatitis involves inflammation of the pancreas, and it may influence blood sugar levels and require hospitalization. This is not the kind of condition you are going to get from moderate drinking, heaving drinking, usually in an acute episode is what triggers pancreatitis.

Heavy alcohol consumption can also reduce the effectiveness of diabetes medications. This can include oral medications, as well as insulin. Consuming large amounts of alcohol in one sitting can lead to rapidly changing blood sugar levels, rendering standard insulin doses ineffective. Alcohol can also directly interfere with the action of many diabetes medications by slowing down their impact.

The use of illegal drugs can trigger type 2 diabetes in some cases and can interfere with the management of type 2 diabetes or prediabetes if you have these conditions. The stimulant drug cocaine is known to directly interfere with carbohydrate metabolism, and so ingesting cocaine on a regular basis can lead to difficulties if you are already having problems managing your blood sugar. Heroin is known to directly interfere with the production of insulin and glucagon by the pancreas, and so it can have an impact on the development or progression of type 2 diabetes. Ecstasy or MDMA is also known to have an impact on blood sugar levels can carbohydrate metabolism.

In short, any abuse of drugs can be bad for those who are prone to prediabetes or type 2 diabetes. The abuse of drugs may even contribute to the development of the disease. Of course, if you are concerned about your health enough to be reading a book about blood sugar and diabetes, it seems likely that you would care enough about your health to avoid the use of illegal drugs and that you will only consume alcohol in moderation.

If you are prescribed one of the legal medications known to possibly trigger type 2 diabetes, discuss your risk with your doctor. In addition, you may want to keep close tabs on your blood sugar in order to avoid the development of problems and spot them as early as possible. If it is possible to use an alternative medication, it is advisable that you do so.

Sleep and Type 2 Diabetes

Getting a good night's sleep is one thing that is becoming recognized as being important to health. Sleep seems to have a large impact on the hormone levels in the body, and it is important for cleaning out the brain and keeping us healthy, not just well-rested. One area that appears to be impacted by the amount of sleep we get appears to be our blood sugar.

Studies are starting to demonstrate with increasing clarity that those who are chronically sleep-deprived are at higher risk of developing many different medical conditions. One of these is the development of diabetes. It isn't entirely known why this is the case, but it is known that the amount of sleep you get each night, and the quality of the sleep that you get, has a major impact on the levels of different hormones, including cortisol, insulin, and glucagon. Some of the impacts of sleep on health may be direct, but they can be indirect as well. In particular, it is known that people who sleep less and have lower quality sleep tend to gain weight more easily, especially over long time periods. Since obesity is directly associated with the development of type 2 diabetes, sleep can influence your susceptibility to developing the disease in this way.

It is important to focus on the importance of the quality of sleep and not just focus on the quantity. Putting the body into a deep sleep seems to be important for avoiding health problems. Different people will need different amounts of sleep in absolute terms, so the quality of the sleep is more important than saying that you need 8 hours of sleep a night. Simply put, many people don't need 8 hours of sleep a night, provided that they are getting quality sleep in 6 or 7 hours per night.

Insomnia is a major factor in determining the quality of sleep. Unfortunately, many people are more likely to develop problems with insomnia as they get older. If you find that you are suffering from insomnia, try to minimize potential causes. Obviously, stress is a major cause of insomnia. It can be generated by all kinds of stress that we all face throughout our lives. Difficulties in relationships can cause one to lay awake at night, tossing and turning. Financial problems usually lead to insomnia, and difficulties at work can cause it as well. If you are having problems with mental stress that are leading to insomnia, you should work on ways to deal with stress more effectively, such as using meditation, and if possible, by directly attacking and solving the problems that are causing you to have stress in the first place. Getting a good night's sleep is so important to your health, that this cannot be overemphasized.

Also, take a look at your sleep environment. If your sleep environment is not comfortable, this can cause problems with insomnia. Is your mattress comfortable and in good condition? Is the room too hot or cold? Factors like these can prevent you from getting a good night's sleep, so it is important to deal with them as best as you are able. Make sure that you have the proper temperature in your bedroom that allows you to sleep comfortably, and make sure that your bed is not making you uncomfortable or causing pain.

Also, watch out for the electronic gadgets. These can interfere with sleep, but sadly we are becoming too addicted to them. Start with the television. It is better to shut it off as opposed to falling asleep with a bedroom television on. You might even consider whether or not you should have a television in your bedroom at all, even though this is a common pastime. Our smartphones and tablets create even more problems. The electrical energy and simple presence of these devices can prevent you from having a good night's sleep, but people are taking them to bed to read electronic books, play video games, or check up on the news and email. One way that is sure to disturb your sleep is to have a smartphone in bed with you, and then you are constantly feeling the tug of checking emails and text messages. Any time that you are trying to fall asleep, and then you get the thought to check for messages, you are going to put the brain back into a heightened state, making it even harder to fall asleep.

Bad sleep habits can directly contribute to the development of diabetes. However, they can contribute indirectly, as well. The more time you spend awake during the night when you should be sleeping, the more likely it is you are going to be feeling hunger pains. This can lead to overeating, and one of the things that is sure to cause weight gain is to eat during the night. Over a long period of time, if you maintain habits like these you are more likely to gain significant amounts of weight, and that can lead to the development of type 2 diabetes. So one thing you should consider is what you are doing with your gadgets, and maybe you might think about leaving them in another room and ignoring them when it's time to sleep. Turn them completely off to reduce the temptation.

Are you overweight or obese?

Being overweight or obese is definitely something that can trigger the development of type 2 diabetes. The more overweight we become, the more insulin resistant our bodies become, and this, in turn, creates a self-feedback cycle. That is, you put on even more weight.

Body fat seems to alter hormone imbalances, and it helps promote problems related to glucose metabolism. Your cells are going to be more resistant to the insulin made by your pancreas. When you become overweight or obese, you also put fat directly on and in the liver and pancreas, and that can inhibit your body from properly functioning.

The role of your weight is so important to the development of type 2 diabetes, that losing weight can be one way of reversing the condition. If you have developed type 2 diabetes and you are overweight, you should consider losing weight as your most important goal. It may even be more important than maintaining healthy blood sugar levels over the short term because if you are able to lose significant amounts of weight, you might be able to get rid of type 2 diabetes altogether. The manner used to lose weight isn't as important as the weight loss itself, but studies are beginning to show that low carb and ketogenic diets are particularly suitable for losing weight when it comes to prediabetics and those with type 2 diabetes. This makes sense because chances are if you develop type 2 diabetes as a result of gaining a significant amount of weight, that means that your body is particularly sensitive to the consumption of carbohydrate contained foods. As a result of this, eliminating carbohydrate-based foods is a surefire way to remove the original problem, and this will trigger weight loss. In turn you will find that over time your blood sugar levels improve, often quite dramatically.

Diabetes Makes you Dramatically Worse Off Healthwise

To understand the impact that type 2 diabetes has on health, it can be instructive to compare the fraction of diabetics having certain health problems to the fraction in the general population. The massive increase in the incidence of various major health problems, if you have type 2 diabetes, and it isn't managed, brings home the seriousness of the disease. Let's have a look at some of the more common conditions that people can develop.

- Kidney Disease: In the general population, about 6% of people will develop chronic kidney disease. Among untreated type 2 diabetics, nearly 28% develop kidney disease. Chronic kidney disease is a very serious health problem that can even be fatal, and if it's not fatal, you might find that you need dialysis to get by.
- Stroke: Stroke is commonly related to high blood pressure. In the general population, the incidence of stroke is 1.8%. Among diabetics, the incidence of stroke is 6.6%. Put another way, a diabetic is more than three and a half times more likely to have a stroke.
- Heart attack: While the incidence of heart attack among the general population is about 2%, among diabetics, it's nearly 10%, depending on the reference. That means a diabetic is 4-6 times as likely to have a heart attack.
- Chest pain: This condition, also known as angina, is closely associated with heart disease and quality of life since it can be debilitating. In the general population, about 1.7% of people report having angina, while 9.5% of diabetics suffer from it.
- Sores/Infections/Amputation of feet: Among the general public, the figure is 10%. Among diabetics, 24% have these problems.
- Serious Eye Problems: Major eye diseases and conditions, including blindness, are prevalent among diabetics that have not gotten proper treatment and achieved suitable management of their condition. In fact, about 19% will develop serious eye damage. The amount in the general public is negligible.
- Congestive heart failure: If you come down with this condition, it is invariably fatal unless you get a transplant. About 1% of the general public deals with this. Among diabetics, the figure can rise as high as 8%.

These statistics make it clear why controlling high blood sugar is important. The incidence of many conditions is much higher among diabetics. When it comes to cancer, research has shown that for most cancers, diabetics are at an elevated risk of developing cancer as compared to those in the general population.

If you are reading this book and you have high blood sugars, but you have not yet been diagnosed with diabetes, you can see the importance of getting your blood sugar under control as quickly as possible. If medication is necessary, you should take the medication, but it is better to do it using diet, exercise, and lifestyle if possible. The role of weight loss will be very important in determining your future health.

Chapter 6: Treatment and 21-Day Meal Plan

In this chapter, we are going to discuss a self-treatment plan to help you manage your own diabetes or high blood sugar problems. It is important to recognize that this is only a suggestion. As we have emphasized repeatedly, you should choose a diet that works best for you, and one that you enjoy. So this meal plan is not something that you must follow; it is merely an example. Some people might choose to follow it; others will find that a different approach is more suitable for their lifestyle and body type.

We are also going to discuss exercise and supplements. There are even a few supplements that can help you to control blood sugar, but in some cases, those will not be necessary. Let's get started by looking at a 21-day meal plan.

Healthy Eating to Control Blood Sugar

As we have discussed earlier, there are several different eating approaches that can be used in order to develop a healthy diet to control your blood sugar. The ketogenic diet is one of the most effective diets for this purpose, and I highly recommend it, having done it myself. However, many people find it too restrictive, and so in this section, we are going to look at a standard low glycemic diet. By consuming low glycemic foods, over the long term you can build up more healthy blood sugar levels and reduce insulin resistance. For some people this can mean reversing diabetes entirely, as long as the diet leads to weight loss. Whatever dietary plan you choose, be sure to pick one that you find is enjoyable and sustainable. A diet that is not sustainable is not one that is going to be producing results.

When following a diet based on low glycemic foods, the most important factor is to watch your portion sizes and also focus on balanced meals. Each time you eat, look to include moderate portions of protein, lots of good fats in the form of olive oil and avocados or fatty fish, vegetables, fruits, and whole grains. Try and avoid snacking, as this can keep insulin levels elevated throughout the day.

A low glycemic meal plan does not mean you have to give up favorites, but you are going to substitute low GI foods for high GI foods when it's possible. As a simple example, substitute sweet potatoes for regular white potatoes, and avoid adding brown sugar and other sweets to the dish.

21-Day Meal Plan

The following meal plan can help you get started with a low glycemic index diet.

Week One:

- Sunday: Breakfast – smoked salmon with half an avocado. Lunch – Turkey sandwich on whole-grain bread, with orange. Dinner – grilled chicken breast, medium sweet potato (butter only), and asparagus.
- Monday: Breakfast – Buckwheat pancakes with blueberries. Lunch- Tuna and celery sandwich with an apple. Dinner – Pork loin, steamed broccoli, and ½ cup whole grain pasta.
- Tuesday: Breakfast – Scrambled eggs with whole-grain toast. Lunch – Sweet potato and corned beef sandwich with Apple. Dinner – baked salmon with spinach stir fry and sweet potato.
- Wednesday: Breakfast – Scrambled eggs with smoked salmon. Lunch – Roast beef sandwich, with orange. Dinner – Trout with salad.
- Thursday: Breakfast – Glass of whole milk with whole-grain muffin. Lunch – Tuna sandwich with 1/2 cup cottage cheese. Dinner- Grilled Turkey burgers, using whole grain buns.
- Friday: Breakfast – Apple bircher Muesli cereal. Lunch – Ham sandwich on wholegrain oat bread. Dinner – Grilled swordfish, wild rice, and ½ sliced avocado.
- Saturday: Breakfast – Quinoa Porridge. Lunch – grilled chicken breast, orange, and Greek yogurt. Dinner- Grilled chicken breast, whole grain couscous, with salad.

Week Two:

- Sunday: Breakfast – Over hard egg on whole-grain toast. Lunch – sliced rye bread with smoked salmon. Dinner – pan-fried lamb steak, couscous, and asparagus with strawberry dessert.
- Monday: Breakfast – Avocado toast. Lunch – smoked trout sandwich with apple. Dinner – Grilled grouper with wild rice and stir-fried spinach.
- Tuesday: Breakfast – Scrambled eggs with one slice of bacon. Lunch – sardines with diced avocado. Dinner – Spicy beef stir fry with whole grain rice.
- Wednesday: Breakfast – Steel cut oats with milk. Lunch – tuna falafel and tabbouleh salad. Dinner – Spicy chicken kabobs with mushrooms, red onion, and bell pepper, and couscous.

- Thursday: Breakfast – Muesli cereal with blueberries. Lunch – Turkey sandwich on whole-grain bread, with orange or apple. Dinner – one pan skinless chicken thighs, with wild rice, sliced tomatoes and peas, and carrots.
- Friday: Breakfast – Scrambled eggs, whole-grain toast, and an Apple. Lunch – Chicken sandwich with avocado slices. Dinner – Chicken salad.
- Saturday: Breakfast – Grapefruit and strawberries with a glass of milk. Lunch – Roast beef sandwich. Dinner – shrimp tacos, with avocado, tomato, red onion, and spicy chili pepper or jalapenos.

Week Three:

- Sunday: Breakfast – Greek yogurt apple muffins. Lunch – Turkey and roast beef sandwich with kalamata olives. Dinner – Pasta with tomato sauce and turkey meatballs.
- Monday: Breakfast – Two eggs, sunny side up, with blueberries and raspberries. Lunch – Shrimp salad. Dinner- Yellow saffron rice with grilled chicken breast and asparagus.
- Tuesday: Breakfast – Cranberry and raspberry smoothie. Lunch – Tarragon chicken and black beans. Dinner – Teriyaki chicken stir fry.
- Wednesday: Breakfast – Feta cheese and tomato 3 egg omelet. Lunch – shrimp and udon noodle soup. Dinner – stuffed peppers with ground bison, quinoa, and lemon.
- Thursday: Breakfast – Perfect scrambled eggs. Lunch – Chicken and black bean burrito, using whole grain tortilla. Dinner – Herb chicken and meatball soup.
- Friday: Breakfast – Fruit salad with banana, strawberry, and blueberries. Lunch – Tuna Sandwich with avocado slices. Dinner – stir-fried chicken, cashew nuts, cubed sweet potatoes, and pearled couscous.
- Saturday: Breakfast – Bowl of whole-grain cereal and milk. Lunch – Greek yogurt. Dinner – sliced roast beef with carrots and broccoli, with serving of whole-grain couscous.

Supplements that can control blood sugar

There are many supplements that can control blood sugar, and they are available over the counter, without the need for a doctor's prescription. I am only going to mention the supplements that have the most scientific evidence behind them for efficacy. The first of these is cinnamon. This common spice is well-known for controlling blood sugar. The best way to take it is in pill form so that you are able to get the dosages that are required in order to have an impact. It is important to know that there are two types of cinnamon, and you want the Ceylon cinnamon. The reason is that the other type can cause bleeding. In fact it is used to make the blood-thinning drug warfarin. If you stick to Ceylon cinnamon, you will be getting true cinnamon that does not have blood-thinning effects, while still getting the benefits that come from its blood sugar lowering properties.

The second over the counter supplement to try is called berberine. Many studies have shown that berberine has a measurable impact on blood sugar management, and if a high-quality berberine supplement is taken on a regular basis for a prolonged time period, it can manage blood sugar as well as prescription drugs like metformin. Berberine appears to increase the number of insulin receptors on cells, thereby reducing insulin resistance. Berberine has been studied mostly in China, and the long-term health impacts of taking it on other body systems are not well understood, but it is believed to be generally healthy. Like metformin, it may reduce the risk of many cancers.

Note that berberine can have real and powerful blood sugar-lowering effects. If you are taking metformin, you should use extreme care when taking berberine, since combining them can lead to a hypoglycemic episode. You should speak to your doctor if you are already taking metformin or other diabetic drugs before taking berberine.

Taking supplements is a personal decision, and supplements can help to enhance the efficacy of your other efforts. However, I prefer to avoid relying on any type of pill, even if it is not prescribed. I am not going to discourage you from using cinnamon or berberine, but my preference is to use diet and exercise if possible. In my opinion, if you are finding that a low glycemic diet is not controlling your blood sugar in the way that you would like, you should try restricting your carbohydrate intake before considering taking supplements or other drugs.

Exercise

Exercise is a very important part of managing your blood sugar. You should seek to exercise at least five days a week, and your exercise should include a mix of aerobic exercise and strength training. Choose the type of exercise that you enjoy doing. You should do aerobic exercise at least 30 minutes per session five days a week. Strength training can be done three days a week. Make sure that you keep your exercise fun; this will ensure that you keep up with it. For aerobic exercise, rebounding is a fun and excellent choice. Swimming, biking, and jogging will work as well. If you live near mountains or wilderness areas, consider taking up hiking.

Simple walking for 30 minutes can also go a very long way toward promoting health. You can also mix up many different exercise activities; there is no reason to restrict yourself to just one method of exercise.

Conclusion

Thank you for making it through to the end of *Blood Sugar*, let's hope it was informative and able to provide you with all of the tools you need to achieve your goals whatever they may be.

Controlling our blood sugar is one of the most important factors in our overall health. Failure to do so not only leads to the development of type 2 diabetes, but it puts us at risk for a wide range of conditions and serious diseases. Among these are heart attack, stroke, and cancer. If your blood sugar gets out of control, you might also find that you develop problems with your eyesight, and you might even go blind. Kidney problems and kidney failure are also more likely – far more likely – among those with diabetes. And we haven't even touched on the propensity of diabetics to develop problems with foot sores and other problems that can lead to the amputation of a foot or even a limb.

The standard view of the medical establishment is that diabetes if you develop it, is inevitable and unstoppable. They also believe it is irreversible and progressive. While the view is slowly changing, most doctors continue to hold onto this viewpoint. Their belief system is based around the idea that if you develop diabetes, the goal is to manage it as best as possible while believing in the background that eventually you are going to lose your battle with the disease, and over time things are going to get worse and worse. Your life will start off with very strict diet recommendations (that are often wrong), together with oral medications and admonitions to engage in exercise activity. Over time, the dosages of your drugs will be increased, and you might find that more drugs will be added to your regimen. It will become harder to maintain your blood sugar in healthy ranges, and you might start experiencing health problems. Eventually, the standard medical procedure is to put you on injectable insulin, and your life will be a constant roller coaster, as you try and manage your disease with injections and pills and constantly worrying about eating.

But does it have to be this way? The good answer is that it certainly doesn't! In today's world, there is enough knowledge and information available to consider a different course of action. You can finally take control over your own health, and it is possible to deal with diabetes using completely natural methods that are often more effective than those offered up by the medical establishment and the big pharmaceutical companies, who like it or not, earn profits by getting people addicted to pills and insulin.

That isn't to say that if you are diagnosed with diabetes, you should not be taking your medication for the time being. But the tools you need to reverse course and possibly get off the medication are there.

The first step in your journey is awareness. This entails knowing what your blood sugars are and how your body responds to the consumption of different foods. You should also face reality and acknowledge problems in your life that may be having an impact on your health. Are you avoiding exercise? Are you overweight or obese? If so, you need to deal with these problems, and these are not problems that you can put off. You need to start attacking them now before it's too late.

Once you understand where you are, by having a clear picture of your blood sugar and A1C results, and admitting your weight problems if you have them, it is time to start taking action to reverse course. Begin by changing your diet. There is not a diet that is suitable for everyone, so you should choose the eating style that works best for your personal tastes, body, and situation. Many readers will benefit the most from a keto diet, while others will do well with a diet focused on balanced meals made from low glycemic foods. If one diet plan is not working for you and producing results, then change to another one. Whatever path you decide to follow, be sure to give it time. A minimum of 90 days should be used with a given diet plan to determine how it impacts your weight and blood sugars. Get support if you need it; no matter what diet you pursue you are going to need to stick to it. Cheating on a diet is only going to put you right back where you started.

The second part of your journey should include exercise. The key is not to focus on doing the most intensive or painful exercise, but to find something that you like doing. It has been shown that most of the benefits of exercise come from the initial activity; in other words, you will get nearly as much out of walking 30 minutes as you will out of running. As a result, don't force yourself to do something that you hate doing. If you don't enjoy the exercise you are engaging in, you are not going to stick to it. But you can't get away from the basic facts; exercise plays a major role not only in the development of diabetes but also in controlling it or reversing if possible. It is unlikely that you are going to be able to manage it without some form of regular exercise.

The third leg of your plan is managing a balanced lifestyle. This means making sure to reduce or manage stress and getting a good nights' sleep. The more research that is done, the more doctors are finding out that sleep is important, and this is true for diabetes. You can help keep your hormones in proper balance – and hence manage your blood sugars more effectively, if you are getting good sleep in the right amounts.

Also, manage your lifestyle by keeping up with social connections and avoiding the problems that come along with substance abuse. If you are abusing alcohol or illegal drugs, get outside help and get rid of your addiction. Failing to maintain a healthy lifestyle by engaging in substance abuse will at best make your blood sugar problems worse, and it could even trigger diabetes or cause other health problems.

Also, look at the prescription drugs that you are taking. If you find that you are taking drugs that can influence blood sugar and possibly trigger diabetes, talk to your doctor about alternatives, or even getting off the medications altogether.

Blood sugar problems, in particular, a diagnosis of type 2 diabetes, can be an earth-shattering event. Get support from family and friends, and also from others who have the condition if you need help dealing with it. There are many online and Facebook support groups you can join to talk with others going through the same things you are. This will help give you the emotional support that you need in order to deal with the diagnosis. You might also get tips and information that will help you manage your condition more effectively.

Sticking with your plan is one of the most important things to remember. Those who develop a plan, even if it is very impactful are not going to succeed over the long term. Those who develop a modestly successful plan that they can stick to for the long term are going to find that they are in better health down the road. Of course we hope that most people can adopt a plan that is both maximally impactful and something that people can stick to overtime. But this is why picking a dietary approach and exercise activities that you like can be just as important as the ability of a specific diet or exercise to control and manage blood sugar. Do what works for you.

If you are having trouble staying motivated, just remember all the pills, needles, and drugs that are going to be necessary if you just follow the standard medical advice. Imagine getting away from all those pills and needles. Taking a natural approach will help you avoid medications or get off the medications if you are already on them. And who wouldn't want that for lifelong health and a long-lived life?

Finally, if you found this book useful in any way, a review is always appreciated!

Madison Fuller

Printed in Poland
by Amazon Fulfillment
Poland Sp. z o.o., Wrocław

57916642R00045